The BMA guide to

PESTICIDES CHEMICALS AND HEALTH

Published on behalf of the British Medical Association by

Edward Arnold

A division of Hodder & Stoughton

LONDON   MELBOURNE   AUCKLAND

A report from the BMA Professional
Scientific and International Affairs
Division.

Project Director: Dr John Dawson

Editor: David R Morgan

Consultant Writer: Robert Gann

Contributors: Dr Len Hutton
Dr Erik Millstone
Dr Tristram Wyatt

Editorial
Secretariat: Tara Lamont
Allison Franklin
Audrey Porter
Sallie Robins
Debbie Pluck

Graphics: Hilary Glanville
Taurus Graphics

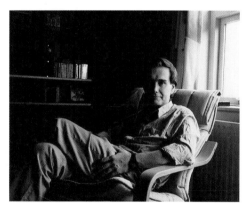

Pamela Taylor

This book is dedicated to Dr John Dawson,
Head of the British Medical Association's
Professional, Scientific and International
Affairs Division (1981–1990), who died on
20 December 1990.

Acknowledgements
Thanks are due to the following copyright
owners for permission to reproduce their photographs.

Friends of the Earth
   (G Beardall and Stephen Lloyd)
Mike Gilchrist
Ms Hilary Glanville (BMA)
Dr Alistair Hay
Henry Doubleday Research Association
Mr Peter Hurst
Dr Len Hutton
Mr Roy Johnson
Mr Alan Johnston
Dr Peter Lemin
The Mansell Collection
Nicaragua Solidarity Campaign
Teaching Aids at Low Cost
Transnational Information Exchange,
   Amsterdam (Chris Pennarts)
Transport and General Workers Union
University of Reading Institute of Agricultural
   History and Museum of English Rural Life
University of Southampton Library Perkins
   Collection
Vincent Wildlife Trust/Nature Conservancy
   Council Bat Project
Which? Way to Health/Adrian Hobbs,
   Consumer's Association Ltd.
Mr Clive Yeomans

First published by British Medical Association 1990
This edition published by Edward Arnold 1992

British Library Cataloguing in Publication Data

Pesticides, chemicals and health.
  I. British Medical Association
  363.17

  ISBN 0-340-54924-6

Typeset in Linotron 202 Baskerville
by Rowland Phototypesetting Limited, Bury St Edmunds, Suffolk
Printed and bound in Great Britain
for Edward Arnold, a division of Hodder and Stoughton Limited, Mill Road,
Dunton Green, Sevenoaks, Kent TN13 2YA by Butler and Tanner Limited,
Frome, Somerset

CONTENTS

INTRODUCTION: BACKGROUND

In July 1988 the Annual Representative Meeting of the British Medical Association (BMA) requested the Council to consider 'pesticide toxicity in the UK, with particular reference to the effects on human health'. In November of that year the BMA's Board of Science and Education agreed that a Working Party should be set up to prepare a report which would cover the health effects of pesticides, with particular reference to food and water. This approach was approved by the BMA Council in January 1989 and the Pesticides Working Party commenced work that same month.

For the purposes of the report it was agreed that the term 'pesticides' should include fumigants, fungicides, herbicides, insecticides, rodenticides and other chemicals used as selective poisons. Pesticide is therefore a broader term than 'insecticide', but does not include other agricultural chemicals such as nitrate.

It is often the place of the medical profession to explore the risks to human health, so that avoidable hazards can be minimized or eliminated. General practitioners and hospital doctors have an important role to play in contributing to the protection of public health from hazards of toxic chemicals. It was clear that information and guidelines were needed by doctors, so that they could advise and counsel patients who might have serious concerns or misperceptions about chemicals and toxic substances.

The pesticide debate, of course, represents part of a wider public concern about environmental pollution in general. A survey conducted by the Department of the Environment in 1989[1] revealed that almost 80% of those polled were concerned about present levels of pesticides, fertilizers and other chemicals in use. These same concerns prompted an enquiry by the House of Commons All-Party Agriculture Committee[2] and an earlier report on agriculture and pollution by the Royal Commission on Environmental Pollution in 1979[3]. Release of the Chairman of the Agriculture Committee's Report coincided with the publication of the Department of the Environment's report on nitrates in drinking water.[4] Other public worries from environmental matters have emerged over the past few years, such as the disposal of toxic waste, and pollution caused by the discharge of untreated sewage into the sea.

The role of pesticides is examined in Chapter 1, tracing the history of their use from ancient to modern times and placing them in an ecological context. In Chapter 2 their place in and influence on the environment is examined, in the context of other pollutants of the soil and water. In Chapter 3 their manufacture and formulation is described, with an outline of current testing procedures. In Chapter 4, the various areas of use of pesticides are reviewed, from agriculture and forestry through to domestic use in the home and garden.

The main subject of this enquiry is the effects on human health. Most evidence relates to exposed populations, such as manufacturers in pesticide plants or farmers and other users of the substances. However, there is also concern about the effect of low level exposure – principally in the food we eat and the water we drink – to consumers and the community at large. The epidemiological evidence relating to the effects of pesticides on individual human health is discussed in Chapter 5 and the risk to the general public health is assessed in Chapter 6.

The use of pesticides is covered by a welter of laws, rules and regulations, and they are outlined in Chapter 7. The need for education and training in the use of these toxic chemicals is reviewed and stressed in Chapter 8, and in Chapter 9 the many and varied ways in which pests can be controlled are described.

The final chapter summarizes the Working Party's review of the actions that need to be taken by the scientific, political, economic, agricultural and industrial communities regarding chemicals and their use.

During the course of the report's preparation, over 200 documents were reviewed relating to every aspect of pesticide exposure. However, despite the extensive nature of this evidence, many questions still remain unanswered. There are many important areas of toxicological and epidemiological research that are not currently available or do not exist. This paucity of scientific data is not, however, in itself an argument for inaction. This report was first published in October 1990 and set out the facts as they were known at that time. Since preparation for publication in this form a number of initiatives and developments have occurred, many of which support the BMA's view that the benefits of the use of pesticides must be balanced against the risks to the public health and environment.

This volume was prepared under the auspices of the Board of Science and Education of the British Medical Association. The members of the Board in September 1990 were as follows:

Dame Rosemary Rue (President, BMA).
Dr A. Macara (Chairman, Representative Body, BMA).
Dr J. Lee-Potter (Chairman of BMA Council).
Dr J. A. Riddell (Treasurer, BMA).
Sir Christopher Booth (Chairman, Board of Science and Education).
Professor J. P. Payne (Deputy Chairman, Board of Science and Education).
Dr J. M. Cundy.
Dr A. Elliott.
Dr R. Farrow.
Dr M. Goodman.
Dr L. P. Grime.
Dr J. F. Milligan.
Dr D. Milne.
Dr G. M. Mitchell.
Dr D. Parry.
Dr M. J. G. Thomas.

The members of the Pesticides Working Party were:

Sir Christopher Booth – (Chairman), Chairman, BMA
Board of Science and Education.

Dr B. M. Buckley – Consultant Physician. Consulting
Toxicologist, West Midlands
Poisons Unit.

Mr P. Hurst – National Health and Safety
Specialist, Transport and General
Workers Union.

Dr J. K. Inman – General Practitioner.

Dr G. M. Mitchell – Consultant Toxicologist. Member,
Board of Science and Education.

Mr A. J. Lees – Water Pollution and Toxics
Campaigner, Friends of the Earth.

The Association is pleased to acknowledge the specialist help
provided by a number of outside experts and organisations
and it is particularly grateful to Dr J. Bonsall, Professor
A. Dayan, Dr A. Hay, Dr R. D. Hodges, Dr L. Hutton, Dr E.
Millstone, Dr A. Watterson and Dr T. Wyatt.

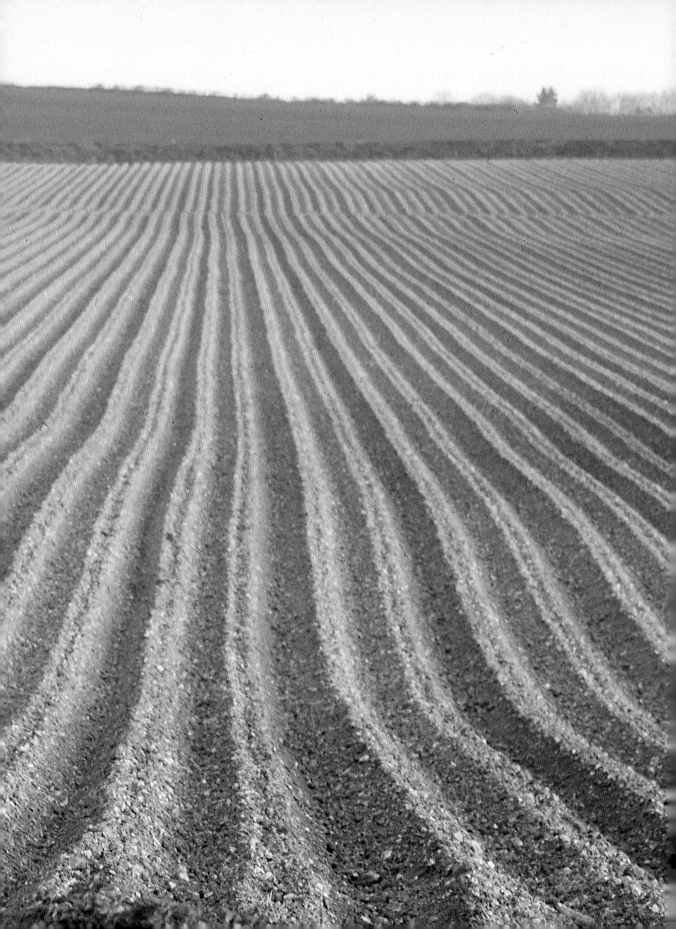

1 THE DEVELOPING ROLE OF PESTICIDES AND OTHER AGROCHEMICALS

MANAGING THE ENVIRONMENT

For centuries people have sought to control their environment. However, it is only in recent times that their attempts to create safe and comfortable living conditions, and to grow plentiful supplies of food, have had anything more than a marginal effect upon the world in which we live.

Vast tracts of the earth's surface were once covered with forests. The demands of a growing population exerted increasing pressure on the earth's resources and more and more land was taken into cultivation. At the height of the Roman period in Britain perhaps 2 000 000 acres (809 000 ha) were under cultivation – a considerable proportion of the more easily cultifiable land then available[5]. There followed a period of decay in the Dark Ages. Recovery began under the Anglo Saxons who made many clearances of forest land for cultivation. The manorial system of the Normans gave farms to the lords of the manor and the monasteries. On some of these farms, especially the monastic ones, there were improvements but generally the system was static. The manor was a self-sufficient economic unit, where the inhabitants possessed what could be obtained from natural resources and fashioned by their own efforts. Tar, furs, iron, spices, silks and fine cloths were recorded as being imported to the manor; but salt, necessary for preserving meat for winter storage, was the only essential item that had to be brought in from outside[6].

In medieval times there was no expectation that people could shape their own environment. The slings and arrows of the natural world were viewed in an essentially fatalistic way. There were areas in which the farmer could rely on his own technical competence – in reaping or milking, for example. But

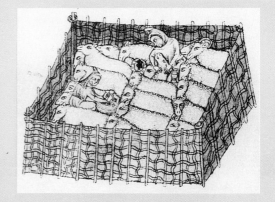

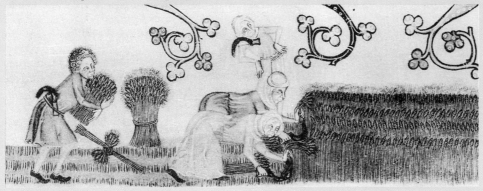

Medieval farmers relied on their own skills in many areas of husbandry and agriculture.

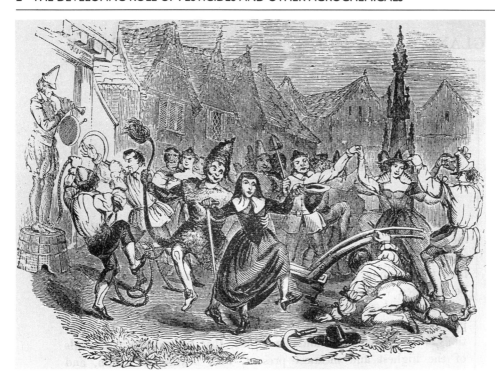

The 1781 Plough Monday Dance of Bessie and the Clown was believed to help crop growth.

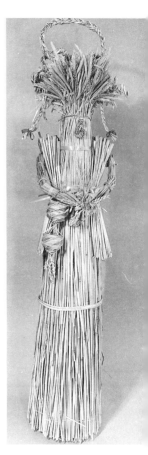

Corn dolly.

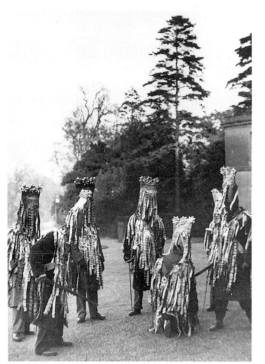

Mumming was a well-established custom, usually practised during the Christmas season.

when he was dependent on circumstances outside his own control (the fertility of his soil, the health of his animals, the ravages of pests or the vagaries of the weather) he was likely to accompany his labours with magical precautions. Keith Thomas's book *Religion and the Decline of Magic*[7] records the existence of a wide range of traditional rites and seasonal observances: Plough Monday to ensure the growth of crops; wassailing to bless the apple trees; Rogation processions and midsummer fires; corn dollies at harvest time. Care was taken to time such tasks as sowing corn or cutting trees to harmonize with the phases of the moon or some other propitious factor. In the absence of effective pesticides there were charms to keep weeds out of corn and magical formulae to deter mice and rats[8].

The decline of magic corresponded with a marked improvement in the extent to which the environment became amenable to control. In several important respects the material conditions of life took a turn for the better during the late seventeenth and early eighteenth centuries. There were significant agricultural improvements, which brought an increase in food production. Increased imports were used to keep down food prices in times of dearth. The growth of overseas trade and the rise of new industries created a more diversified economic environment.

In the 1720s Daniel Defoe undertook his tour through England and Wales[9]. The impression of English agriculture left by Defoe is one of enterprise and experiment. Stress was laid on fertilizing the soil. On Salisbury Plain sheep were folded on newly ploughed land to manure it. In Cheddar where 'the whole village are cowkeepers, they take great care to keep up the goodness of the soil by laying on large quantities of dung for manuring'. All this was before what is usually regarded as the age of the Agricultural Revolution, and already close links were beginning to develop between agriculture and industry. Wheat passed from the farms to the corn millers, bakers, distillers, and starch makers. In the form of flour it was used by stationers, book-binders, printers, trunk makers and paper-hangers. Barley went to the distilleries, but its chief industrial use was to make malt and hence beer. Sheep provided wool for the English textile industry and cattle provided hides for tanners and hence leather for a variety of trades. The fat of both was used by soap and candle makers, the horns by cutlers, and the bones by glue manufacturers[10]. 'Agribusiness' had arrived.

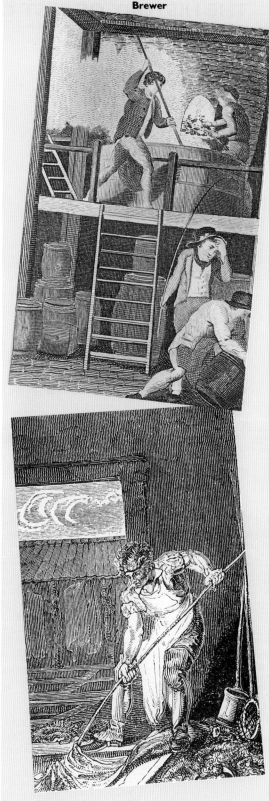

Brewer

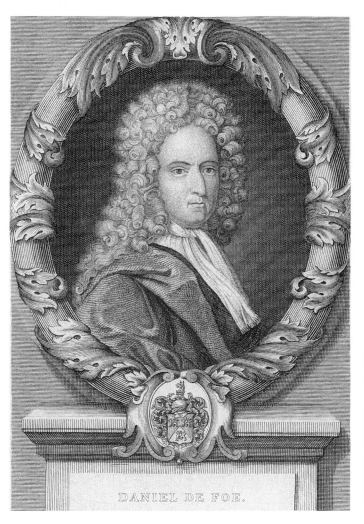

Daniel Defoe

DANIEL DE FOE.

Tanner

THE HISTORY OF PEST CONTROL

The evidence of history shows that in previous centuries the mass of the population suffered terrible diets and chronic shortages of food, because of crop failures, pest damage and adulteration (as well as deliberate policies such as land clearance, and the basic condition of poverty). The account in the book of Exodus (10: 12–16) of the plague of locusts in Egypt is early testimony to the havoc that insect pests can cause, and which is experienced still by people in the African continent. The widespread contamination of rye crops up to this century by the fungus ergot is believed to have caused the mass outbreaks of delirium known as St. Anthony's Fire[11]. The widespread use of pesticides to combat these problems is not found until the twentieth century, although references to the use of chemicals in agriculture may be found well before this. Homer mentioned the use of sulphur in fumigation in 1000 BC. Democritus was aware of insecticides in 470 BC and used olive extracts on plants to prevent blight. In 200 BC Cato was using sulphur fumes to destroy vine pests, while the Romans used the plant hellebore to control rats and mice. Pliny in the period AD 23–77 knew about fungicides, and in his *Historia Naturalis* advocated the application of wine to cereal seeds to prevent mildew. The ancient Chinese understood biological control and used ants as predators to protect trees from insect pests, but by AD 900 they were also using chemical methods, with arsenic, to control garden insects. Dried chrysanthemum flowers, of the type that are used to prepare the natural insecticide pyrethrum, have

Chrysanthemum flowers contain a natural insecticide.

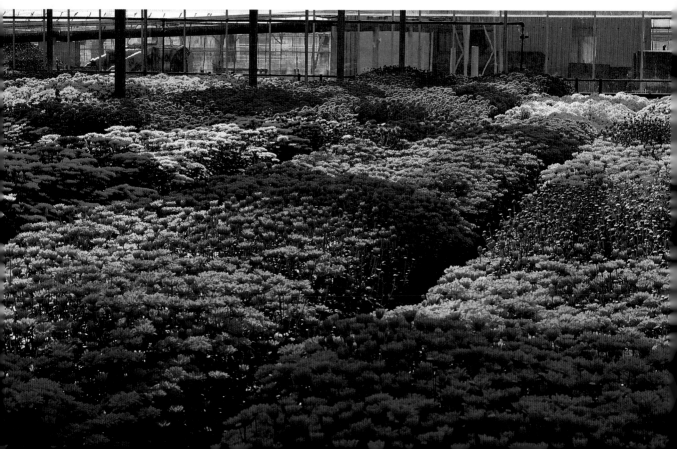

been used since at least the last century to kill pests on food crops. Similarly plant root extracts, such as derris, which are used in insecticides today, have long been used to paralyse river fish in traditional fishing techniques. But the development of chemical methods of pest control only really started in the mid-nineteenth century and then was slow to become widely established. The earliest chemical pesticides were for the control of insect pests, but subsequently preparations were developed for the control of weeds, fungal infections and, more recently, for other competitive organisms and to control the ripening process[12].

A visit to the Perkins Collection of early agricultural books at the Hartley Library, Southampton University offers a fascinating insight into early use of pesticides. The use of urine, soap suds, tobacco, lime and, *in extremis*, arsenic recurs throughout the agricultural books and pamphlets of the eighteenth and nineteenth centuries. *The Complete Vermin-Killer* of 1775 advocates 'juice of henbane infused in strong vinegar for green bugs', and 'for caterpillars, an equal quantity of the lees of oil and the urine of an ox'. The remedy for ants shows a concern for possible adverse environmental effects: 'mix some powder of arsenic with honey, put it into a box made of card, pricked full of holes with a bodkin. Be careful not to make the holes too large, lest bees should likewise get in and be poisoned'. For those who are cautious about the use of arsenic a robust alternative is offered: 'laying a quantity of human ordure on the anthills occasions pismires to leave the place'.

William Forsyth was the king's gardener at Kensington and St. James' and in this capacity carried out a number of experiments on fruit trees. His *Treatise on the Culture and Management of Fruit Trees*, published in 1802, includes a substantial section entitled 'Observations on the diseases, defects and injuries in all kinds of fruit and forest trees'. Forsyth mixed his preparations on a large scale: for example, a lime water potion for use against red spiders and aphids. A suspension of 'two bushels and half a peck of lime in 550 gallons of water' was made up in 'a cistern seven feet long, three and a half feet broad and three feet deep.' The mixture was sprayed onto fruit trees by means of a 'barrow engine, pressing your forefinger over the mouth of the pipe to spread the water like the falling of small rain.' Spraying should be done in cloudy weather, when there is no danger of frosts or wind from the north or east. Forsyth also counsels caution in the use of arsenic: 'I would advise never to use arsenic or corrosive sublimate (for rats and mice) except under particular circumstances, for they are deadly poison.'

It is evident from the number of editions that there was considerable interest in contemporary manuals on pest control. Benjamin Holdich's *An Essay on the Weeds of Agriculture*, first published at the turn of the century, was in its fourth edition by 1825. Holdich largely advocated preventive measures: drainage, weeding, burning and fallowing. But he clearly had a keen interest in less laborious methods:

'An enlightened agriculturist, T. B. Evans, informs us that common salt dropped on the crown of sainfoin effectually destroys it, without injury to the crop of grasses. Children may be employed to apply the salt by hand to the weeds; and

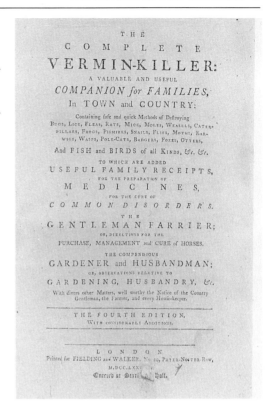

Title page of the eighteenth-century work *The Complete Vermin Killer*.

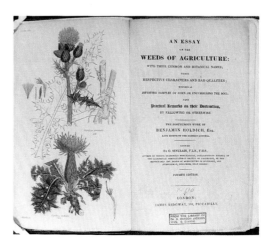

Pages from *An Essay on the Weeds of Agriculture*, by Benjamin Holdich.

THE

ENGLISH GARDENER;

A TREATISE

ON

THE KITCHEN GARDEN, THE FLOWER GARDEN,
THE SHRUBBERY, AND THE ORCHARD.

WITH

A KALENDAR,

Giving Instructions relative to the Sowings, Plantings, Prunings, and other
labours, to be performed in the Gardens, in each Month of the Year.

BY WILLIAM COBBETT.

"I went by the field of the slothful, and by the vineyard of the man
void of understanding ; and, lo ! it was all grown over with thorns, and
nettles covered the face thereof, and the stone-wall thereof was broken
down. Then I saw and considered it well ; I looked upon it, and received
instruction."—Proverbs : chap. xxiv. ver. 30.

LONDON AND GLASGOW:
RICHARD GRIFFIN AND COMPANY.

**Title page of the nineteenth-century work *The
English Gardener***

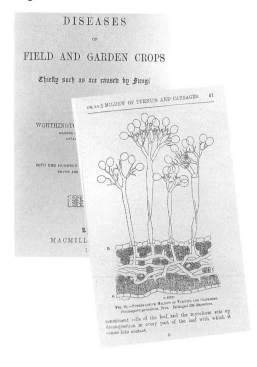

**Illustration from the 1884 manual *Diseases of Field
and Garden Crops* by Worthington Smith.**

when we consider how much more expeditiously and safely
the remedy may be used in comparison to pulling up the
weeds by the roots, it is doubtless a valuable discovery.'

The English radical and farmer, William Cobbett, recorded
his frustrations in dealing with pests in his *English Gardener*
(1829). He felt powerless when dealing with ants, and also had
an early perception of the blunderbuss action of non-specific
pesticides:

'I know nothing but fire and boiling water, or squeezing to
death, that will destroy ants; and, if you pour boiling water on
their nests in the grass, you destroy the grass; set fire to a nest
of the great ants, and you burn up the hedge or the trees, or
whatever else is in the neighbourhood. As to squeezing them
to death, they are amongst the twigs and roots of your trees
and plants; they are in the blossoms, and creeping all about
the fruit; so that, to destroy them in this way, you must
destroy that also which you wish to protect against their
depredations.'

But Cobbett also made use of some of the principal techniques
of integrated pest management, including the encouragement of
natural predators.

'Lime has no effect upon caterpillars, and your only hope is
that your other enemies, the sparrows, will lend their assistance in delivering you from these; and I do verily believe,
that, were it not for the sparrows, and other birds, these
insects would make it next to impossible to cultivate gardens
in England.'

Experimentation with agricultural chemicals developed during
the latter part of the nineteenth century, although there was
little effect on everyday farming practices. Agriculture continued in the normal, traditional manner. This could be described as 'organic' today, but whereas modern organic
agriculture – although based on traditional systems – has
matured in a way that ensures that crops grown in well-run
organic farms are anything but vulnerable[13], in those days
crops were still highly susceptible to attack by pests and disease.
For example, the Irish potato crop was ruined by potato blight
in the 1850s, and millions starved or were forced to emigrate[14].

The discovery of the effects of sulphur to control powdery
mildew on vines 150 years ago provides an early illustration of
how chemicals were being used to control pests. Indeed,
milestones in the history of pesticide development have long
tended to coincide with outbreaks of a particular plant disease
or pest attack, as Hubert Martin pointed out in 1928 in his
work, *The Scientific Principles of Plant Protection with Special Reference
to Chemical Control*[15]. Bordeaux Mixture (copper sulphate and
lime), originally used to stop children from stealing grapes, was
introduced in 1882 to counter the 1879 outbreak of vine downy
mildew; Paris Green (copper arsenite) in 1867 to control the
spread of Colorado Potato Beetle which had occurred in the
1850s; and prussic acid (hydrogen cyanide) in 1886 for the
control of scale insects in fruit trees.

The 1884 manual *Diseases of Field and Garden Crops* by Worthington Smith provides a good picture of pest management

towards the end of the nineteenth century. Like Holdich almost 100 years before, Smith provided sound advice on prevention (buying good quality seed, practising scrupulous crop rotation and burning any diseased crops) and there is little mention of the possibility of using chemical fertilizers. A rare exception is the recommendation for dealing with bunt in wheat seed: 'The seed should be washed or steeped in some weak poisonous solution – sulphate of soda in a weak solution – and the seeds afterwards dried with dusted quicklime.' During the 1880s and 1890s there is, however, the beginnings of the technology of pesticide application, with E G Lodeman's *The Spraying of Plants* (1886) describing various types of knapsack sprayers, steam powered sprayers and complex nozzles.

Fifty years on, beyond the First World War and its stimulus for scientific and industrial endeavour, a new story arises. H. C. Long, a Ministry of Agriculture scientist, was a prolific pamphleteer and writer of articles in the agricultural press. His 1934 pamphlet *Suppression of Weeds by Fertilisers and Chemicals* is as interesting for the wealth of advertisements for pesticide and chemical fertilizer products as it is for Long's own thesis. There was by then a thriving agrochemical industry, with different companies competing for custom from farmers. Prominent among the advertisers was ICI Fertilisers. Others included the Nitrate Corporation of Chile ('Suitable manuring may so stimulate cultivated crops that many of the worst weeds will be crowded out'), the National Sulphuric Acid Association ('a quick simple and safe method of cleaning a crop: suitable for spraying under almost all weather conditions') and Cyanamide ('supplies nitrogen and lime to the soil and has caustic properties which are of great value in agriculture for weed destruction and the control of numerous pests').

Up to the Second World War, however, the chemical control of pests rested on very few substances. These were mainly inorganic compounds such as copper and mercury salts, and elemental sulphur, for use as fungicides, and general poisons such as arsenic and cyanide, for insect pests. Organic compounds included by-products like tar distillates, and plant extracts such as derris, nicotine and pyrethrum. Few of the pesticides available at that time were targeted at particular pests, and selectivity was largely a matter of timing of application. Most were highly toxic and dangerous to use. Their use was confined mainly to high value produce such as fruit, hops, market garden and glasshouse crops[3]. Towards the end of the 1930s the insecticidal properties of DDT were recognized, and were to be exploited dramatically in controlling the louse vector of human typhus, and later in the control of the mosquito vector of malaria. In the early 1940s the potential for broad-leaved weed control using phenoxy acid derivatives was being realized.

The modern agrochemical age has developed largely since the Second World War. The period of rapid increase in the availability and use of modern pesticides began with the introduction of the insecticides DDT and HCH, and of the hormone-type herbicides 2,4-D and MCPA in the late 1940s, and the organochlorine pesticides dieldrin and aldrin in the 1950s. These became objects of widespread public interest in the 1960s: DDT, dieldrin and aldrin through the publication of Rachel Carson's *The Silent Spring*[16], and 2,4-D with the related

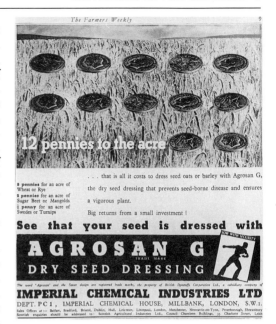

A pesticide advertisement from the 1930s.

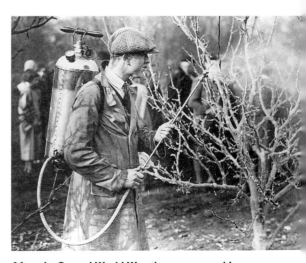

After the Second World War there was a rapid increase in the availability and use of pesticides particularly DDT.

2,4,5-T through their extensive use as defoliants by the US forces in Vietnam.

The first moves towards controls over pesticide use in the UK came in 1950 with the Working Party on Precautionary Measures Against Toxic Chemicals Used in Agriculture. Chaired by Professor Solly Zuckerman, the Working Party succeeded another committee – the Gower Committee – which had advised that protective clothing should be made compulsory for all farm workers using toxic chemicals. Zuckerman and his colleagues soon became convinced of the need for a coherent system of statutory controls over the manufacture and use of pesticides. However, the Ministry of Agriculture, Fisheries and Food (MAFF) rejected the concept of statutory controls as being 'an unwarranted interference with the freedom of commercial concerns' and instead brought in the voluntary Pesticides Safety Precautions Scheme[17]. Statutory controls over pesticides did not come into force in the UK until 1986, with the Control of Pesticide Regulations (made under the Food and Environment Protection Act 1985).

A DEVELOPING TERMINOLOGY

The term 'pesticide' is of comparatively recent origin. The *New Oxford English Dictionary* (2nd edition) gives the first recorded use of the word as recently as 1939, with the establishment of the Pesticides Supply Committee. In September 1943 the *Farm Journal and Farmer's Wife* was observing that 'a new word "pesticide" has crept into the garden literature this year.' 'Pestology' has an earlier pedigree. The word was first used in the *Daily Express* of 23 September 1927 where there is an early observation on the excesses of some enthusiasts: 'The pestological exhibition and conferences opened yesterday. There were insect powders, sprays and pastes, and this will show you how far a pestologist goes – automatic firearms!' The more specific terms 'herbicide' and 'insecticide' are of earlier origin. 'Insecticide' was first used in 1871. At this time it had no particular chemical connotation, and the first usage in the *Encyclopaedia Brittanica* referred to 'the starling's character as an insecticide makes it the friend of the agriculturist.' By 1894 *The Times* was able to comment on the current availability of 'spray pumps and other insecticidal apparatus'. The *Vermont Agricultural Experimental Station Annual Report* provides the first use of the term 'herbicide' in 1899 – 'carbolic acid is a valuable herbicide but the herbicidal action is of short duration.'

The term 'pesticide' was not used in *Index Medicus* (the index of medical literature produced by the US National Library of Medicine) until 1948, although 'insecticide' appears much earlier in 1908. The earliest reference so far traced, in a French publication, shows an interest in the adverse effects of pesticide use on human health[18].

In the UK the legal definition of pesticides under the Food and Environment Protection Act 1985 is 'pesticides and substances, preparations and organisms prepared or used for the control of pests or for protection against pests; and for correct purposes.'

In 1947 *The Times* reported 'the demand for Gammexane

pesticide is growing rapidly'. But by 1958 the seeds of doubt were beginning to be sown, as the *Manchester Guardian* commented, 'chemical weedkillers should be used only as elements in a management programme, not as specific pesticides to use when weeds become a nuisance.' *The Times* of May 1969 declared that 'the chief threat to birds of prey is pesticides.' By 1971 *Power Farming* was stating that 'Shell, like most other companies in the field, recognise that indiscriminate use of pesticides is highly undesirable.'

THE NEED FOR PESTICIDES

Pesticides have played an important part in the dramatic increases in agricultural productivity which have been achieved in the developed world over the last few decades. The contribution to the eradication of the pests which destroy crops and spread disease has been considerable. There has been much investigation of the gains in crop yields that may be attributed to the use of pesticides. These can readily be demonstrated under controlled experimental conditions, but are more difficult to assess in 'real life' usage where the position is complicated by other factors, for example the introduction of higher yielding plants and heavier use of fertilizers.

In evidence to the 1979 Royal Commission on Environmental Pollution[3] the British Agrochemical Association (BAA) provided figures for the amounts by which the yields of some crops would theoretically be reduced if pesticides were not used. The figures were based on surveys carried out in 1975 and 1976 and suggested that the cereal crop would be reduced by 24% in the first year and 45% in the third. The loss in the first year would be due to pest damage, while the increased loss by the third year would be due to a build up of weeds. In 1967 it was estimated that, on a world scale, 30% more food, cotton and other crops could be available if they were not destroyed by pests[19]. More recently, the International Group of National Associations of Pesticide Manufacturers (GIFAP) has made similar claims: 'Even with modern cultural techniques, at least 30% of the world's potential crop production is lost each year. Crop losses would be doubled if existing pesticide uses were abandoned'[20].

A 1989 Food and Agriculture Organisation (FAO) report[21] estimated that losses from pests and disease in the field are 20–40% of the crop worldwide and may be higher in developing countries. Losses continue at almost every stage of the chain leading from field to table: during harvesting, drying, storage, milling and cooking. The average level of loss here has been estimated as 10% for grains and grain legumes, and 20% for less easily preserved crops such as roots, fruit and vegetables.

In its series of briefing papers *Pesticides in Perspective*, published in 1987, the BAA provides a number of answers to the question 'Why use pesticides?' These can be summarized as follows:

1 *Improving food quality* – It is assumed that consumers want to buy food that is unblemished. Through the use of pesticides the UK's farmers and growers are able to fill

shops with produce that is clean and of good quality, at reasonable prices. Although some people have an understandable desire to eat 'natural food', it is hard to demonstrate differences in taste, nutritional value, or healthiness between food grown with the use of chemicals and that grown organically. There is some evidence of improved food quality from organic systems, particularly in relation to its nutritional value[22]. On the other hand, a 1990 Consumers' Association Survey found that gourmets and lay people alike had difficulty in differentiating between food grown organically and food grown with the use of chemicals.

2 *Reducing food prices* – The success of modern farming, has meant that the percentage of its income that the average family spends on food continues to fall. In 1985 a pound of potatoes cost 45% less, allowing for inflation, than it did in 1975. The use of pesticides and fertilizers, as well as advances in plant breeding and husbandry, has made a significant contribution to this situation.

3 *Maintaining public health:* Disease-bearing insects and rodents are a hazard to health, particularly in hospitals and catering establishments. In the Third World in particular, people in large geographical areas are at risk from insect-borne diseases such as malaria, sleeping sickness, plague and Weil's disease. (Some fungi contaminate food and produce dangerous toxins, some of them highly carcinogenic to man.)

4 *Promoting animal welfare* – Insecticides can give substantial relief to a range of problems, for example from the irritation caused by flies, to maggots which can literally eat sheep alive. In cattle, blindness and gangrene of the udder can be prevented.

5 *Banishing drudgery* – Hoeing and hand weeding is backbreaking, monotonous and exhausting. In developing countries it can take up most of the waking day for men, women and children. Herbicides offer an escape from drudgery, but this can be a mixed blessing. On some large plantations in the Third World agricultural workers are losing their jobs because of the use of pesticides.

6 *Aiding habitat management* – Herbicides can play a useful part in the management of wildlife habitat, for example in controlling scrub. They are used by the Nature Conservancy Council and in public gardens, parks and sports grounds. Water companies and local authorities use pesticides to control aquatic weeds without damage to fish.

7 *Earning export revenue* – Last and perhaps not least, pesticides are big business. In 1985 total sales of pesticides amounted to almost £900 million. About 60% of this sum was accounted for by exports, making an important contribution to the balance of payments.

PUBLIC ATTITUDES

The publication in 1962 of Carson's *Silent Spring*[16] was the first popular expression of a growing concern about the indiscriminate use of pesticides, more specifically dichloro-diphenoltrichloroethane (DDT), dieldrin and aldrin. DDT was first synthesized in the nineteenth century, but introduced on a large scale to agriculture in the USA in the 1940s. In 1955 the World Health Organisation (WHO) started a worldwide malaria eradication programme using DDT, estimated as having saved 15 million lives by 1965 and continuing today. Research in the 1960s was beginning to suggest that DDT was carcinogenic in mice and, although DDT was never shown to be harmful in man, in 1971 it was banned in the USA. In Britain it was subject to a voluntary ban from 1974 to 1984, when it was removed from the market.

Dieldrin and aldrin were not completely banned in the UK until 1989. Some of the hazards arising from the use of dieldrin and aldrin (which degrades to dieldrin) are illustrated by the results of a survey of dieldrin residues in eels, undertaken by the Government in 1986. This revealed a higher level of dieldrin than set out in the Acceptable Daily Intake (ADI) in eels from many of the sampled rivers in the UK, including all the sampled English rivers. The Government's Committee on Toxicity of Chemicals in Food, Consumer Products and the Environment noted the Government's recommendation that 'those people who regularly consume eels caught in those areas where contamination is highest should be advised to restrict their intakes.'[23]

DDT provides the classic example of a problem that faces governments, the agrochemical industry, and the medical profession. Environmental groups, however, point to the fact that in many areas the mosquito species that carry malaria are exhibiting a high level of resistance to DDT, thus rendering it largely ineffectual for malaria eradication in those areas. Friends of the Earth (FoE) also point to evidence from the Solomon Islands where the use of DDT to control mosquitos resulted in the poisoning of lizards which had fed on the dead and dying mosquitoes. Cats, in turn, were poisoned by feeding on the lizards, which were previously too difficult for the cats to catch in large numbers. With fewer cats, there was a population explosion of rats, leading to the widespread use of rodenticides. The effects on owls feeding on poisoned rats have yet to be ascertained but the 'agrochemical' sales were certainly boosted.

Pesticides undoubtedly play their part in the maintenance of public health and availability of plentiful, cheap and consistent supplies of food, here and in the Third World, and a well fed population is much less susceptible to disease. But is this at a cost to the environment and to the health of the population?

PESTICIDES AND THE ECOSYSTEM

This report is concerned mainly with the direct effects of pesticides on human health, but it is now recognized that the overall health of the human species is ultimately dependent

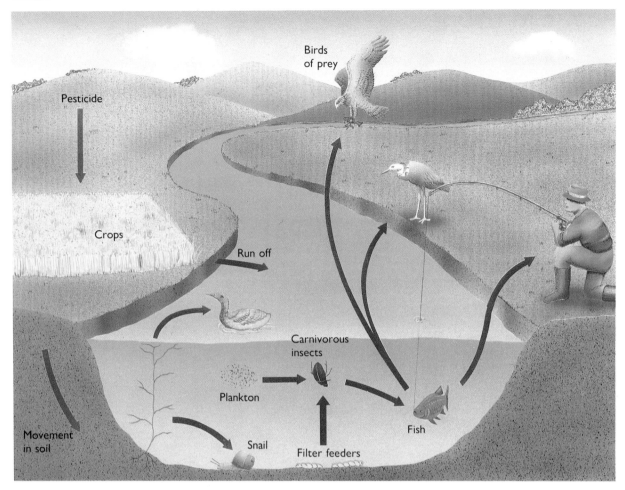

Figure 1.1
Infiltration of pesticides into a food web.

upon the biological system of which we are part. Globally this dependence is becoming increasingly apparent, as the effects of deforestation manifest themselves in climatic change, desertification, and species loss. It is therefore worthwhile at this stage to consider aspects of our ecosystem – a set of interacting, independent living and non-living components or subsystems – and how it may interact with external factors.

Pesticides are necessarily poisonous, at least to some species. Human beings exist only as part of a complex global ecosystem in collaboration with a large number of other species. Any decline in the numbers of a particular species can cause disruption of the ecosystem, with possible long-term effects on humans that are unpredictable. Besides the possibility of their causing the death of certain numbers of species, these chemicals may have subtle effects on the behaviour and physiology of wildlife. The chances of survival and reproductive success of affected individuals could be altered. Obviously these effects are more likely to occur after concentration of the chemical up the food chain. Our present understanding of the environmental impact of pesticide use is incomplete. However, it is clear that the effects of pesticides on human health must include a wider consideration of the interplay between chemicals and the environment.

An ecosystem consists of three nutritional groups: producers (mainly plants) synthesizing organic food by incorporating energy from the sun; consumers (mainly animals); and decomposers (bacteria and fungi). Energy from the sun runs through this system as organisms at each level extract the energy necessary for survival. Thus a food chain is constructed[24].

A simple chain such as this will be a subsystem of a complex macrosystem in which many chains interlock to form a complex web. There are two principal components, a grazing food chain and a detrital food chain, whereby dead plants and animals are broken down by a series of decomposing organisms. In this process of eating and being eaten energy flows through the system, passing from one level to the next. But this energy transfer is not efficient because about 90% of the energy is lost as heat. Therefore each level must eat sufficient quantities of the previous level to maintain life, and there is a finite amount of biomass that can be supported by a given quantity of food[25].

In the human agroecosystem, arable cropping is the most energy-efficient method of providing food. There is minimal loss of energy in this one-step food chain. In contrast, the use of arable crops to feed cattle for human food is much less efficient. This is because of the substantial loss of energy in first converting the plant carbohydrate to animal protein before human consumption. To support a large human population therefore, energy has to be put into the system by, for example, maximizing crop yield by using fertilizer and pesticides. Many of these substances require hydrocarbon (oil) for their manufacture, either as a raw material or energy source. When the quantity of fuel oil consumed by tractors, crop drying and storage, transport and packaging is taken into account, there is often actually a net energy deficit, that is more energy is put into the system than is extracted as food. Ecologists express this scientifically as an 'energy ratio (Er)':

$$Er = \frac{Energy\ (food\ output)\ per\ hectare}{Energy\ density\ (input)\ per\ hectare}$$

In subsistence agricultural systems, the energy ratio may range from 1:0 to 7:0, indicating a high output of food energy in relation to energy input. However, in many industrialized arable systems the energy ratio may be as low as 0:1.

Although pesticides ensure that energy is not diverted along unwanted (for example, weed and insect) food chains, they are inclined to infiltrate other food webs (Figure 1.1) and thereby derange the natural balance.

Creatures lower in a food chain generally reproduce more rapidly and are more numerous than their predators, and they are therefore capable of rapid adaptation by natural selection. In other words, there are successively smaller numbers of creatures (less biomass) at each step up the food chain and predators breed more slowly than their prey. Thus a 'Pyramid of Numbers' is established.

Many general pesticides kill both pests and their predators. For example, insecticides used for killing aphids may kill the ladybirds that prey on them, and surviving ladybirds may starve as aphid numbers are depleted. When a field has been cleared through pesticide application it is usually the pests that increase again at the fastest rate, either through immigration or through breeding from survivors (thereby increasing chances of

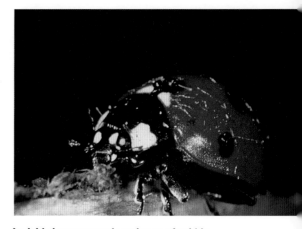

Ladybirds are natural predators of aphids.

induced pesticide resistance). The predators subsequently build up their numbers slowly, and the farmer may discover a 'rebound' phenomenon as the pest reappears, but this time there is reduced predator activity. Sometimes a new 'pest' occurs. A creature whose numbers were previously held in check by competition for food or by other natural enemies may emerge as a major pest; these are called 'secondary' pests. The farmer then sprays again and the pesticide treadmill is established[26].

Pesticide applications may infiltrate biological systems by the process known as bioconcentration (Figure 1.2). Bioconcentration is a characteristic of food chains, whereby substances present in low or insignificant amounts in the environment are concentrated with the ascent of each step in the chain, as predator consumes its prey.

The classic example of this is the non-biodegradable organochlorine group of insecticides (for example, DDT, dieldrin, and aldrin). They are particularly harmful in living systems owing to their high fat solubility and persistence: even after 17 years some soils may retain as much as 39% of the amount originally applied. The concentration of such pesticides has been investigated in aquatic ecosystems. For example, research in California in the 1950s showed the following increase in concentration at each step: from water to plant plankton, 265 times; to small fish 500 times; to fish 75000 times; and to the fatty tissue of grebes 80000 times. From that particular ecosystem, the western grebe was nearly eliminated. Such a process was recently described for dieldrin[23] as affecting eels and herons in England. Any person enjoying a diet with a higher than average intake of eels would be also at risk of exceeding the ADI of dieldrin. Interestingly, substantial bioconcentration of a pyrethroid insecticide (permethrin) was reported as having been observed in a ciliate protozoan, an observation not previously noted for this class of chemical and which may be of great significance for higher trophic levels in the food chain[27].

From the mid-1970s persistent organochlorine insecticides

Figure 1.2
Through a process of bioconcentration minute quantities of chemicals in the environment may be concentrated as they pass up the food chain.

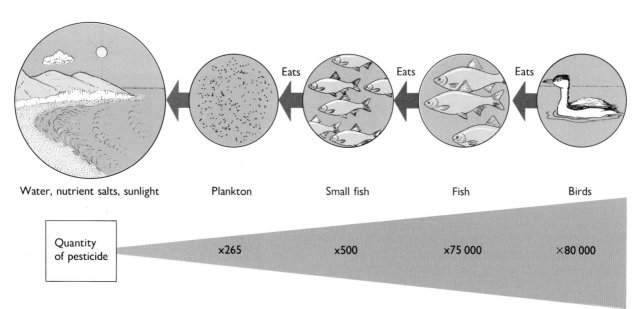

| Water, nutrient salts, sunlight | Plankton | Small fish | Fish | Birds |

Quantity of pesticide — x265 — x500 — x75 000 — ×80 000

have been phased out by regulation, to be replaced by highly toxic but biodegradable insecticides. Biodegradation, the breakdown by micro-organisms of natural and synthetic chemicals in soil and water, reduces the accumulation of pesticide residues in the environment. Without biodegradation, the environmental level of contaminant would rise rapidly to critical levels. Some of these degradation products, however, are relatively stable and may be toxic. For example, gamma-HCH (also known as lindane) degrades in water into the more toxic compounds alpha- and beta-HCH. Generally, pesticides if not leached away are dissipated from the soil by microbial metabolism. A growing body of literature[28] is showing that some pesticides degrade at accelerated rates in soils that are repeatedly treated with the same chemicals. This 'enhanced biodegradation'[29,30] causes rapid inactivation of the chemical and results in ineffective pest control. The phenomenon was first described in 1949[31], and is now well recognized as affecting many pesticides. It occurs because the use of pesticides triggers rapid evolutionary adaptation, not only in the pest which is the target, but also in soil bacteria, micro-organisms, invertebrates and higher plants which are not. Thus exposure to these pesticides causes the genetic selection of individual organisms whose biochemical make-up or behaviour is such that the toxic effects are nullified.

There are many papers about this phenomenon of adaptation, which also leads to pesticide-resistant pests. This may influence pesticide costs and crop yields; pests are mobile and the actions of one farmer may affect others in his vicinity. House flies from factory farms in East Anglia are now resistant to a wide range of insecticides[32].

In 1984 the World Resources Institute reported that 'from the early 1900s to 1980, 428 species of arthropods are known to have become resistant to one or more insecticides or acaricides. Over 60% of these species are of agricultural importance, while the remainder are either pests of medical concern or nuisances to people. Among plant pathogens of agricultural crops, over 150 resistant species are known. An estimated 50 herbicide-resistant weed species have now been reported'[33,34]. The BAA points out that there are over 20000 insect pest species, and of the 428 species mentioned in the survey 'only 20 were of any economic importance'. Research continues to develop more pest specific chemicals which destroy a much narrower range of target species. In addition, alternatives like genetically engineered pest controls are also being developed.

With the steady proliferation of new insecticides and their increasing usage, the number of scientifically documented cases of insecticide resistance has increased considerably[35] (Table 1.1). These figures underestimate the severity of the resistance problem worldwide because the susceptibility of many insect pest species has been studied only partially, or in many cases not at all. In addition, the doubling time for the numbers of resistant species to a particular class of insecticides has decreased over time as each new class is introduced[35] (Table 1.2).

Pests may also become resistant to DDT and the synthetic pyrethroids through a similar biological mechanism, and long established and widespread DDT resistance threatens the efficacy of synthetic pyrethroids[26]. This is because many pests

Year	No. of resistant species
1938	7
1948	14
1956	69
1970	224
1976	364
1980	428
1984	447

Table 1.1
Numbers of documented cases of insecticide resistance

Insecticide class	Average doubling time of resistant pests (years)
DDT/methoxychlor	6.3
Lindane/cyclodienes	5.0
Organophosphates	4.0
Carbamates	2.5
Pyrethroids	2.0

Table 1.2
Doubling time for numbers of species resistant to insecticide

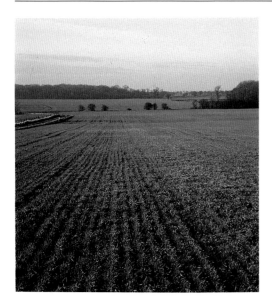

Monoculture, may lead to weed resistance to the herbicide.

have now expressed genes conferring resistance to various classes of pesticide. Such developments of cross- and multiple resistance to a class or classes of pesticides has reduced the efficacy of many chemicals. Fortunately, the problem has been to some extent mitigated by other genetic factors (for example, recessive resistance genes), ecological factors (for example, high immigration rates of susceptible pests) and operational factors (Integrated Pest Management, IPM).

The first reports of herbicide resistance appeared as long ago as 1968[34], and since then numerous reports have appeared in the literature. In particular, these have been associated with so-called 'monoculture'[30] whereby the same crop is grown year after year in the same field without rotation and is usually treated repeatedly with the same herbicide. This results in the induction of tolerance to the herbicide in use; and consequently higher rates of application, the addition of other chemicals, or both become necessary.

Concern is being expressed about further hazards of monoculture. Some scientists believe that plant inbreeding has now weakened food crops so that they are now vulnerable to epidemics. Many of the plant stocks in use today are so-called 'high risk' stocks which, if left to themselves, would neither set nor grow without constant intervention and care. Unlike many pests, these new hybrid varieties are lacking in the genetic diversity necessary for population defence by natural selection and therefore require a heavy pesticide input. When new diseases appear, crop breeders try to find resistance in an absolute line and, if this is not possible, they attempt crosses with wild varieties. Thus genetic engineering, inserting resistance genes, requires extensive plant gene stocks. The problem is that gene 'banks' are not being properly maintained; and, at a meeting of the American Association of the Advancement of Science, plant geneticists expressed anxiety at the inadequacy of international stockpiles of seeds and other genetic materials for food crops. In future years, the use and control of plant genetic resources are due to become major international political and financial issues.

There are also reports of other secondary effects of pesticides, by which we refer to the unpredicted defects of sublethal doses of pesticides on target and non-target organisms. The potential significance of this topic is considerable when one considers all the possible interactions. For example, pesticides may influence the crop itself, either by causing enhancement of, or complete loss of, resistance. Certain fungicides may act by eliciting the plant's natural defences to potential pathogens; such chemical activation of the plant's natural defence system may pose less hazard than synthetic systemic fungicides. The herbicide glyphosphate interferes with the synthesis of certain amino acids in barley, thereby reducing resistance to fungal infection. Study of such interactions is at an early stage, but clearly could have far-reaching implications for understanding the impact of pesticides on crop production and reducing the amounts used.

The application of pesticides to areas adjacent to streams and rivers frequently leads to contamination of these aquatic habitats. Run-off, direct overspray and drift during application may result in concentrations lethal to certain biota. The synthetic pyrethroids are particularly toxic to aquatic invertebrates: zooplankton are important crustaceans, serving as a link within aquatic ecosystems by recycling essential nutrients from biota and non-living matter via consumption and excretion, as well as becoming prey for other fish. Their removal from the aquatic ecosystem therefore may have profound effects on its structure and function.

Contamination of groundwater by agricultural chemicals is becoming a major environmental concern. Worry is centred not only on nitrogen fertilizers, but also on pesticides. The problem is primarily detected in shallow groundwater at present, but chemicals enter aquifer systems to be transported to greater depth. In addition to the obvious relation to amounts applied, this is determined largely by the relative rate of percolation and degradation of chemicals in soil.

The factors affecting the fate of any organic chemical on the soil environment are legion, ranging from soil type (for example, clay content, pH, and water content) through to the physico-chemical properties of the substance (for example, degradation rate, distribution between vapour, solid, liquid and absorbed phases in the soil). Even within a single plant species the uptake varies; there may be local competition in the soil between the organic and other soil solids for the partitioning of organics from solution. More volatile chemicals may, depending on soil type, vaporise and penetrate a plant via foliage as well as roots. The process is extremely complicated and knowledge in this area is constantly being expanded.

There is a well-documented incidence of pesticide residues in water supplies. A survey of levels in England and Wales revealed levels above the Maximum Admissible Concentration (MAC) for any single pesticide in 298 water supplies. The principal contaminants were atrazine and simazine, both used extensively by local councils and British Rail. It has been suggested that this spoiling of groundwater quality might be reduced by employing interceptor ditches to redirect the contaminated water away.

WHO used chemical pesticides to great effect in its global plan to eradicate malaria. However, by 1980, 51 of the 60 malaria carrying mosquito species had developed a resistance to three insecticides – DDT, lindane and dieldrin – which were crucial to the eradication programme. At least ten species were also resistant to the organophosphates malathion and fenitrothion, while more developed resistance to the carbamate propoxur. Eighty-four countries now have malaria mosquitoes resistant to at least one of the major pesticides, and the incidence of malaria is increasing again with a doubling of reported cases between 1972 and 1976. WHO has now withdrawn the use of DDT on environmental grounds.

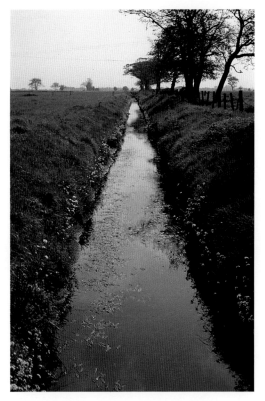

The aquatic ecosystem may be damaged if pesticides inadvertently drain into the waterway.

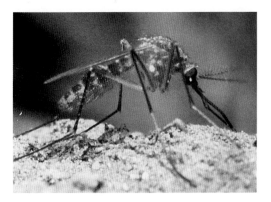

By the 1980s nearly all the malaria-carrying species of mosquito were resistant to the three main insecticides used by the World Health Organisation.

HUMAN HEALTH CONCERNS

The possible impact on the ecosystem is the first of two major concerns about the use of pesticides today; the second relates to worries about the possible impact on the health of the population. Two types of exposure should be distinguished: acute and chronic toxicity.

Acute toxicity is evidenced by almost immediate effects. The route of absorbtion may be through inhalation, through the skin or through ingestion.

Chronic toxicity is present where effects are produced by long-term intake of lower or intermittent doses.

There is concern about five possible outcomes of pesticide exposure:

1 Carcinogenicity (ability to cause cancer).

2 Mutagenicity (damage to genetic material).

3 Teratogenicity (effects on the foetus).

4 Allergy and other effects on the immune system.

5 Effects on the nervous system.

Turning first to acute exposure, there undoubtedly is widespread poisoning from pesticides worldwide. This poisoning can take three forms: attempted suicide, accidental poisoning or occupational poisoning. A 1986 WHO report estimated that there were between 800000 and 1500000 cases of unintentional pesticide poisoning worldwide, leading to between 3000 and 28000 deaths. The figures for acute poisoning include, of course, a spectrum of conditions ranging from minor cases of skin and eye irritation through to serious systemic effects. The figures given for deaths are also tentative, and WHO admit that these are only very rough estimates based on extrapolation from the few countries where records of poisoning do exist. Dudley[36] quoted figures for Sri Lanka indicating that in 1978 over 15000 people were admitted to government hospitals suffering from pesticide poisoning, of whom 1029 died. Seventy per cent of the fatal poisonings were thought to be the result of suicide bids, but this still leaves over 300 accidental deaths. These figures were based on the situation in the early 1970s and take no account of newer, safer pesticides.

The record on acute toxicity in the UK is very much better, and illustrates the importance of proper handling and use. In the period from 1974 to 1986 there was no fatal accident from a pesticide in normal use; in 1987 a fatality arose from the use of a pesticide when a forester illegally used cyanide to destroy a wasps' nest. Turning to domestic use, Government statistics for 1984 reported that 110254 accidents of all kinds required attendance at an accident and emergency department. Only 59 of these involved pesticides, fewer than the number of accidents involving deck chairs and flower pots. In respect of acute toxicity the newer insecticides undoubtedly represent a considerable improvement on many of the older organochlorine, organophosphorus and carbamate insecticides. Also, many pesticide and other chemical incidents causing acute effects undoubtedly are not reported because there is no national incident monitoring scheme comparable with the 'Yellow Card' system, which is used by doctors and dentists to report adverse effects of drugs. The introduction of a similar system for pesticide incidents would be a major step forward, but this would have to be accompanied by clear reporting criteria and the necessary education in the use of the system. At present the various poisoning information centres, the Health and Safety Executive (HSE), MAFF, and industry all collect data on pesticide incidents. While there is good communication between the different agencies, many minor incidents are probably not reported. One way of simplifying this would be to have a single monitoring unit.

The risks to health from long-term exposure are much less clear. Given the extensive use of pesticides, both for agricultural and non-agricultural purposes, it is almost impossible for any member of the population to avoid exposure to very low levels of different pesticides in food and water. Consequently, there is public concern about the possible adverse effects on human health arising from long-term exposure (chronic toxicity).

Cancer is one of the more serious diseases that may be linked to pesticides. To date 49 chemicals, including some pesticides, have been reviewed by the International Agency for Research on Cancer (IARC)[37]. Eleven were found to be possibly carcinogenic or carcinogenic in animals and, although it is difficult to extrapolate from animal studies, there was no evidence that any were carcinogenic in man. However, at the same time the US Environmental Protection Agency (EPA) has been able to establish the harmlessness of only 37 of the 600 active ingredients used in the 45 000 different products currently marketed in the USA.

It is important to remember that no chemical can ever be proved to be totally safe, and that virtually all apparently harmless substances are toxic to man at a sufficiently high dose. Paracelsus, writing in the fifteenth century, recognized this when he said 'Everything is poison, nothing is poison; it is the dose which makes the poison.'

The debate on the health implications of agricultural chemicals is surrounded with uncertainties. It is on these uncertainties that regulatory decisions have to be based. The World Health Organisation in collaboration with the United Nations Environment Programme has supported this view[38] and stated:

"The increasing use of [such] pesticides has lead to widespread concern about their potential ill-effects on human health. The situation is particularly worrying in view of the lack of reliable data on the long-term consequences of exposure to pesticides."

It is tempting to err on the side of safety and to ban any chemical suspected of causing serious health problems but, no chemical, including pesticides, can ever be proved totally safe. As in medicine risks must be balanced against benefits[39].

PRESENT USE OF AGRICULTURAL CHEMICALS

In 1986 Goldsmith and Hildyard produced a report which commented critically on the level of pesticide production and use in the UK[17]:

'In the three years between 1974 and 1977, the area of cereals sprayed with aphicides increased 19 times. Between 1979 and 1982, the area of crops treated with insecticides doubled, while the area treated with fungicides more than doubled. BAA figures from 1979 to 1982 for the five major crops grown in Britain (cereals, potatoes, oilseed rape, sugar beet and peas) show a 29% increase in the area sprayed with herbicides, a 37% increase for insecticides and a 106% increase for fungicides. Yet the actual cropped area only increased by four per cent.'

The 1979 Royal Commission on Environmental Pollution[3] concluded, 'the evidence submitted to us suggests that there is an upward trend in the sales of pesticides which reflects increased usage and not merely increased costs' (Figure 1.3). Sales of pesticides by UK manufacturers for home and export use rose from £30 million a year in the late 1940s to £150 million a year by the mid-1970s. The latest figures from the BAA (1988) show UK sales of over £400 million, together with exports totalling over £600 million (Table 1.3). When inflation is taken into account this means that the value of agrochemical sales has increased by inflation only, and there has been no real growth. Over the same period, the weight of active pesticide ingredients

Figure 1.3
In 1988, domestic and export sales of agrochemicals totalled over £1,000m.

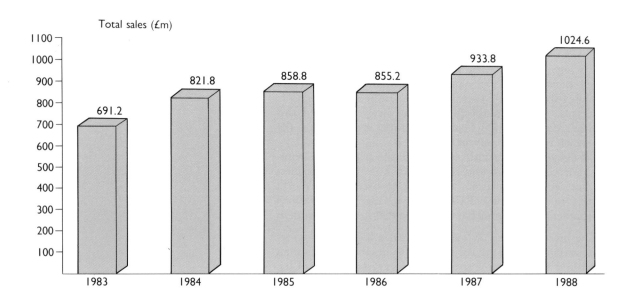

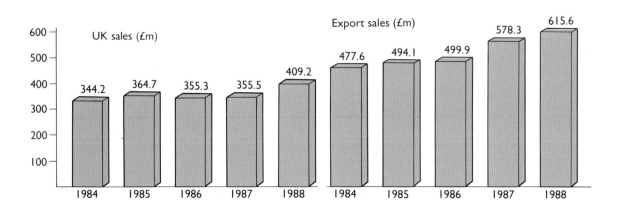

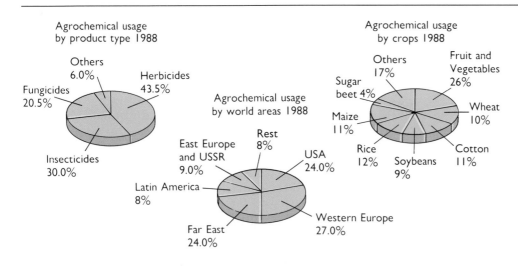

Agrochemical usage by product type 1988

Agrochemical usage by world areas 1988

Agrochemical usage by crops 1988

Figure 1.4
In the developing world insecticides are the most commonly used agrochemical.

Table 1.3
Sales and exports of pesticides in the UK

Area of use	1982	1983	1984	1985	1986	1987	1988	% change
UK sales (£m)								
Herbicides:								
Agriculture, horticulture	146.6	176.6	166.5	174.1	175.8	178.0	201.6	13.2
Industry, forestry	4.2	4.5	4.7	5.6	5.9	6.3	6.9	9.5
Garden, household	7.9	7.6	7.0	6.9	8.6	8.6	10.4	20.9
Total	158.7	188.7	178.2	186.6	190.3	192.9	218.9	13.5
Insecticides:								
Agriculture, horticulture	19.1	25.8	30.9	28.5	25.2	23.4	28.9	23.5
Industry, forestry	0.8	0.4	1.1	0.9	0.8	0.9	1.0	11.1
Garden, household	4.4	4.6	4.6	7.0	5.7	5.7	7.7	35.1
Total	24.3	30.8	36.6	36.4	31.7	30.0	37.6	25.3
Fungicides:								
Agriculture, horticulture	59.3	75.9	90.2	98.1	94.5	97.4	108.8	11.7
Industry, forestry	0.5	0.5	0.6	0.8	0.8	0.9	1.0	11.1
Garden, household	1.0	0.9	1.1	1.4	1.2	0.9	0.8	(11.1)
Total	60.8	77.3	91.9	100.3	96.5	99.2	110.6	11.5
Molluscicides:								
Agriculture, horticulture	–	–	–	–	–	6.9	8.9	30.0
Seed treatment:								
Agriculture, horticulture	8.5	11.5	14.7	17.1	13.8	12.3	11.3	(8.1)
Growth regulators:								
Agriculture, horticulture	3.3	4.6	6.7	7.2	8.8	9.9	11.4	15.2
Herbicides/fertilizer mixtures:								
Garden	1.5	2.8	2.3	1.7	2.3	1.9	3.0	58.0
Other pesticides	10.9	11.3	10.9	12.0	9.4	5.4	7.5	38.9
Total	271.6	329.8	344.2	364.7	355.3	358.5	409.2	14.1
UK exports (£m)								
Herbicides	151.8	214.7	269.9	244.5	253.7	302.4	310.7	2.7
Insecticides	89.2	103.5	138.9	168.0	159.5	171.3	194.8	13.7
Fungicides	18.0	27.0	50.5	64.8	72.7	92.9	90.3	(2.8)
All others	16.3	16.2	18.3	16.8	14.0	14.5	19.8	36.6
Total	275.3	361.4	477.6	494.1	499.9	581.1	615.6	5.9

Source: Reproduced from *The British Agrochemicals Association Annual Report and Handbook, 1988–89*

actually declined from 33 157 tonnes to 23 504 tonnes. At the same time the hectares treated increased from 15.1 million to 19.6 million. The average rate of application of pesticides per hectare has fallen from 2.2 kg to 1.2 kg. This is evidence that the agrochemical industry is making advances in the introduction of products that do the required job at lower dosage rates to the hectare, by targeting pests, weeds and disease with greater accuracy than was possible previously.

Improvements in technical and engineering controls, especially of spraying equipment, are necessary to ensure that users are better protected. Some of the defects in the controls over the use of pesticides, especially for post-harvest treatments, have been highlighted by the Residues Sub-Group of the Government's Research Consultative Committee.

In 1988 the Sub-Group reported that: 'The procedures used for applying the pesticides to harvested produce can vary in their degree of sophistication from the accurate "metering" of the pesticide with mechanical mixing and the use of chemical solutions as post-harvest dips and drenches to ensure a uniform distribution of the active ingredient on the produce, to cruder "bucket and shovel" methods.'[40]

Furthermore, in the case of cereals, the Sub-Group stated that, 'stored produce may also be subjected to repeated pesticide treatment or admixed with freshly treated produce introduced later into the storage container.' In the case of leafy vegetables and root crops, it reported that, 'these are normally treated with fungicides for protection against storage diseases. Methods of application are fairly crude and more work is needed to determine the uniformity of fungicide distribution in relation to the permitted average residue levels.' The Sub-Group concluded that, in consequence, 'the levels of pesticide residues on stored produce leaving the farm gate can vary considerably from batch to batch.'

A global perspective, however, gives a rather different picture. World production of pesticides in 1986 was 2 300 000 tonnes and is now increasing worldwide at a rate of 12.5% a year.

The greatest area of growth in pesticide sales is undoubtedly the Third World. By 1981 33.5% of all pesticide use was in the Third World and the proportion is increasing fast. The figures are even more significant when the use of insecticides is examined (Figure 1.4). Insecticides make up only 28% of the USA's total use of plant protectants and only 20% of European consumption. However, insecticides are by far the most important plant protectants used in developing countries, making up 63% of total pesticide use in Africa, 58% in Latin America and 57% in South East Asia[41]. Insecticides are significant in those countries for two reasons: firstly, insects are the most common pests; and secondly, the availability of cheap labour for hand weeding means that less herbicides are used.

Pesticides are not the only agricultural chemicals that are being used in increasing quantities every year. Scientists from the Water Research Centre, a private company, estimated in 1987 that farmers were using ten times as much inorganic nitrogen fertilizer as they did in 1945. In the late 1930s 60 000 tonnes of nitrogen fertilizer were spread on agricultural land in the UK each year. By 1985 this had increased to 1 580 000

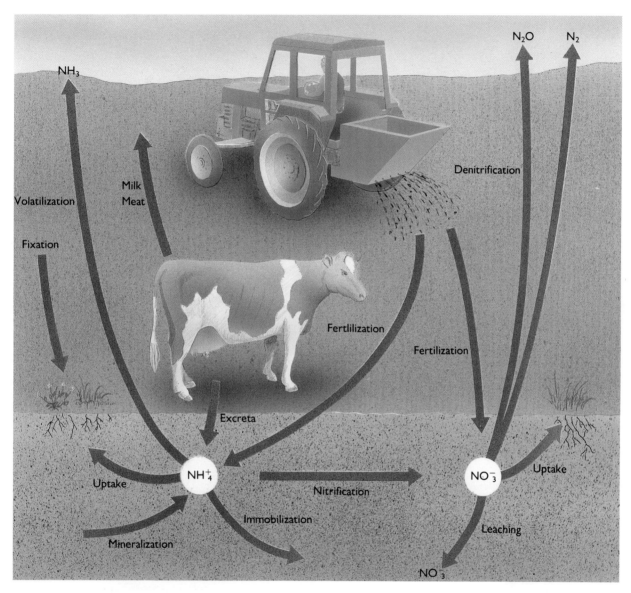

Figure 1.5
The nitrogen cycle

tonnes[42]. Only about half of the fertilizer applied is taken up by the crop. The other half is lost in a variety of ways – by leaching to surface or ground-water, by denitrification to the atmosphere, by combination into the soil's organic matter and so on[43]. The Royal Society's 1983 report on the nitrogen cycle (Figure 1.5) considered that '440 000 tonnes of fertilizer nitrogen are added to arable soils and perhaps as much as 150 000 tonnes of nitrate nitrogen are lost by leaching each year.'[44]

As a result of leaching of nitrates to the water supply an estimated 1 500 000 people in the UK are now exposed to nitrate levels in drinking water exceeding the limit of 50 mg l^{-1} set by the EEC, which is, however, more than the 44.5 mg l^{-1} given in the 1984 WHO guidelines on Drinking Water.

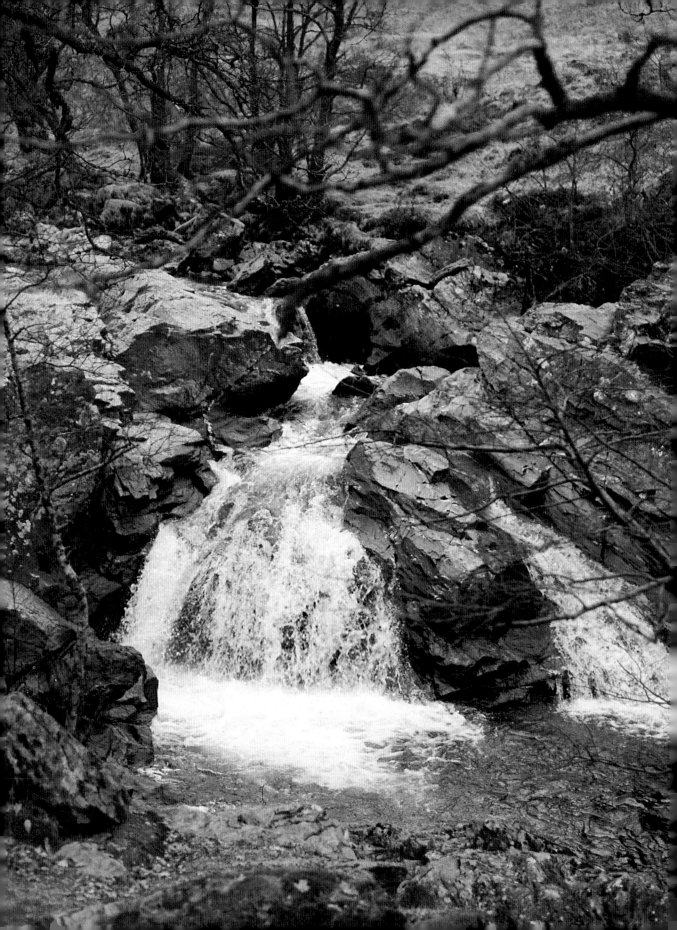

2 PESTICIDES, CHEMICALS AND THE ENVIRONMENT

In assessing the possible risks to health of the public by the use of pesticides, it is necessary to consider other pollutants, both natural and man made, which affect the air we breathe, the food we eat and the water we drink.

We are made up of chemicals; the air we breathe, the food we eat, and the environment we inhabit are all chemical. Early in 1983, the American Chemical Society's Chemical Abstract Service registered its 6 000 000th chemical. The US Toxic Substance Control Act Inventory lists 63 000 chemical substances whose manufacture, processing and ultimate use for commercial purposes has occurred in the USA since 1975. Additionally, the number of synthetic organic chemicals used and disposed of by society is increasing at a rate of about 1000 new chemicals a year[45].

There is a common misconception that synthetically produced chemicals are the ones that are bad for us. In fact, proven carcinogens are to be found in 'natural' foods, such as celery and parsnips (psoralens), mushrooms (hydrazines), basil (estragole), peanuts (aflatoxin), black pepper (piperine) and mustard (allgliso-thio cyanates), to name but a few. Vegetables known to be mutagenic include lettuce, paprika, rhubarb and string beans[46]. Cereals can also be an important source of fungal toxins, such as the ergot fungus. Recently Dr Roger Fenwick of the Institute of Food Research has suggested that society should be concerned equally about all chemicals present in food whatever their origin. Dr Robert Scheuplein, Director of the Office of Toxicological Services at the US Food and Drug Administration, has estimated that 98% of cancer risk in the diet comes from ordinary food, in that natural carcinogens in the diet overwhelm all the others. The human body has evolved to cope with small amounts of a wide range of chemicals every day. The simple ploughman's lunch of bread, cheese, butter, onions and chutney contains 10000 different chemical substances, without including food molecules such as proteins and carbohydrates.

Most known substances have no known effect on health and the environment. Others are moderately hazardous, a number are dangerous and a few are so potentially harmful that they require highly controlled handling and storage. Over recent years increasing amounts of synthetic and natural chemicals have been returned to the environment after use. The original constituents are taken from the environment, their chemical nature altered and the products are frequently widely redistributed. Thus crude oil and gas from Saudi Arabia are transformed into plastic containers, which then litter Europe and North America. Lead mined in Missouri is combined with

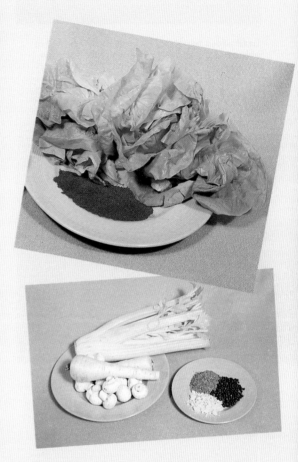

Some everyday foods contain substances hazardous to human health when taken in massive quantities.

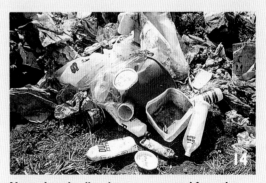

Natural crude oil and gas are removed from the environment and transformed into non-biodegradable products such as plastic.

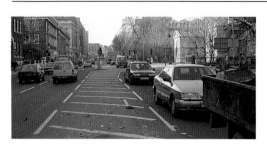

Lead added to petrol is subsequently emitted in exhaust gases causing environmental pollution.

four ethyl groups to make tetraethyl lead, which is then added to petrol to improve its combustion characteristics. Lead is subsequently emitted in exhaust gases and unburnt petrol fumes into the air of every city and town in the world[6]. The effects of many synthetic chemicals on human health, particularly at low exposure levels over long periods of time, are as yet unknown.

If we continue to synthesize chemicals, which will be done if we are to continue with a standard of living to which twentieth-century society has become accustomed, then we face a crisis, not only in their safe use, but also in their safe manufacture and disposal.

THE WATER CYCLE

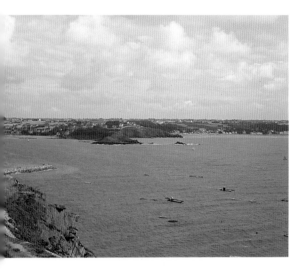

Seawater makes up 97% of the Earth's total water supply.

Only about 3% of the Earth's total water supply is fresh, and the bulk of that is locked up in polar ice caps or as ground-water so deep that it is inaccessible. The remaining 97% consists largely of seawater, with less than 1% in fresh and brackish inland waters[47]. Very nearly all of the world's water was of naturally good quality until the Industrial Revolution in Europe and North America. Industrial technology powered by fossil fuels (coal and oil) and a rapidly increasing rate of urbanisation began the discharge of large amounts of polluting effluent into water supplies. Now the entire water environment, or 'hydrosphere', is contaminated to some degree by human activities.

Water evaporates from the oceans to form precipitation such as rain, snow or hail, which may then fall over land and run off over or through the ground back into the oceans. This process, the water cycle (Figure 2.1), is summarized in the Royal Society of Chemistry's *Understanding our Environment*[48].

Precipitation

Rain, snow and hail are not, of course, pure H_2O. First, they contain atmospheric gases – mainly nitrogen, oxygen and carbon dioxide dissolved from the air. Secondly, they contain solid matter and other substances dissolved from impurities in the air which are derived from the earth's surface – such as sea spray, volcanic emissions and wind-borne dust. Thirdly, they contain ozone and gases derived from chemical reactions, triggered by solar and cosmic radiation, between naturally occurring materials in the atmosphere. Finally, precipitation contains impurities from man-made pollution of the atmosphere, for example sulphur and nitrogen oxides, smog chemicals and particles.

Ground-water

Precipitation passes through the surface soil and underlying permeable strata where many impurities are removed by natural processes. The water continues to move downwards through the unsaturated rocks until it accumulates in saturated, permeable rocks lying over the impermeable rock layer. The saturated, permeable layer in which the water collects is called an aquifer. Large amounts of ground-water may be held in aquifers, which effectively store water in pores in the rock like a sponge (Figure 2.2).

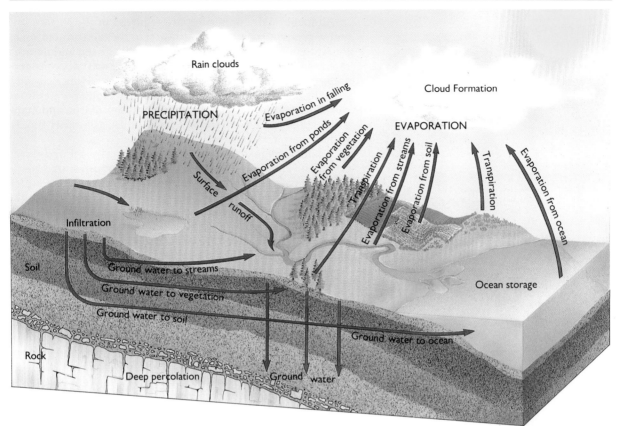

Figure 2.1
The water cycle, driven by the sun, lifts purified water from the land and oceans, to fall again as rain or snow.

Ground-water is often ignored as a water supply resource because it is out of sight, but in England and Wales 28% of the drinking water supply is derived from ground-water (Figure 2.3). The major aquifers in the UK are the chalk regions of the south of England. Other important aquifers lie in the limestone areas of the Cotswolds and Yorkshire, and in the sandstones of the East Midlands.

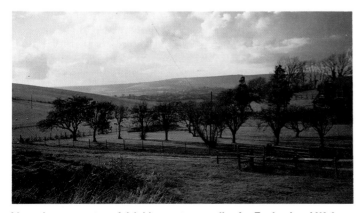

More than a quarter of drinking water supplies for England and Wales are drawn from groundwater filtered through chalk aquifers such as the South Downs.

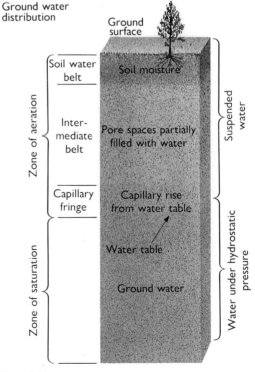

Figure 2.2
Permeable strata and groundsoil act as a filter for groundwater.

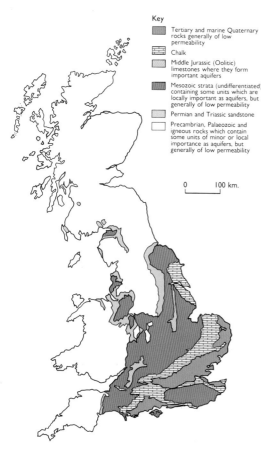

Key

- Tertiary and marine Quaternary rocks generally of low permeability
- Chalk
- Middle Jurassic (Oolitic) limestones where they form important aquifers
- Mesozoic strata (undifferentiated) containing some units which are locally important as aquifers, but generally of low permeability
- Permian and Triassic sandstone
- Precambrian, Palaeozoic and igneous rocks which contain some units of minor or local importance as aquifers, but generally of low permeability

0   100 km.

Figure 2.3
Major aquifers in the UK are formed of the chalk regions in the south of England.

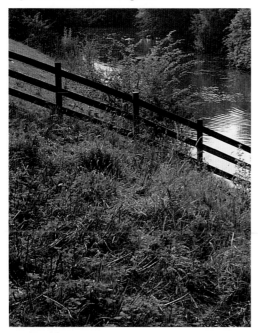

Good quality fresh water can support a wide range of aquatic life.

Although many impurities are removed in the surface soil and vegetation layer and by filtration in the unsaturated zone, the water will also dissolve chemicals from the soil and unsaturated zone. The quality of the resulting water will vary considerably, depending on the particular type of overlying soils and rocks in the aquifer. For example, shallow ground-water from riverside gravels may contain concentrations of iron and manganese high enough to render it unfit for use as a water supply without specific treatment.

While much material is filtered out naturally, ground-water pollution is now a major concern in many industrialized countries. One of the problems is the very slow rate at which water moves through an aquifer, generally less than a metre a month. Once contaminated, an aquifer may retain pollutants for years. Hence the importance of protecting the ground-water from pollution in the recharge area. It is also very difficult and takes a long time to clean up an aquifer once it has been contaminated. Additional costs will be incurred for treating extracted water that has been polluted.

Freshwater streams, rivers and lakes

The quality of stream, river and lake water reflects the quality of the upstream contribution of surface run-off water and ground-water. However, these waters, open to the energy of sunlight, also become the media for the growth of living things – aquatic biota. These biota can be divided into phytoplankton (plants, mainly algae, which float with the water); zooplankton (bacteria, protozoa, and other minute animals); rooted plants, growing from the bed of the stream or lake or floating in the water; and larger animals, which either swim freely or are attached to plants or the bed of the stream. The nature, variety and balance of these biota are determined not only by the natural environment, but also by man's intervention such as the construction of dams and weirs and, of course, chemical pollution.

Rivers and streams rely on aquatic biota to break down organic wastes washed into them, provided there is sufficient dissolved oxygen in the water to enable the biota to live and breed. So rivers can purify themselves if organic waste is adequately diluted (Figure 2.4). The amount of oxygen dissolved in the water depends on the rate of exchange with atmospheric oxygen which, in turn, is strongly dependent on temperature. The lower the water temperature, the more oxygen is dissolved in the water. Streams and rivers at 10°C contain about 10 mg l^{-1} of dissolved oxygen. If a clean river suddenly receives too much organic waste, the initial effect is that the number of biota also proliferate given a potential increase in food supply. But the increased number of organisms will then use up all the dissolved oxygen in the water and, unable to breathe, will die. The river will become smelly and septic because there are no biota left to break down the waste.

Estuaries

In a tidal estuary there is a gradual change from freshwater to the saltwater state. The boundary at which a river becomes an estuary is usually called the tidal limit. This is the furthest location up river from the sea where the water level is noticeably

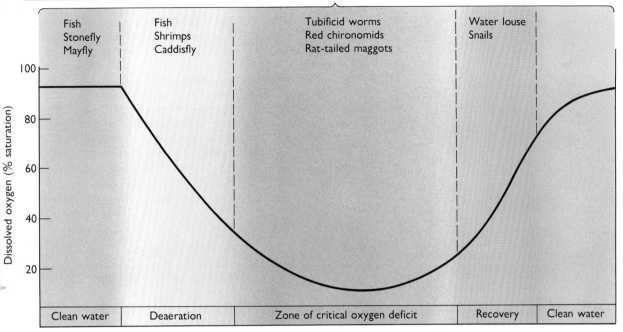

Typical composition of aquatic community

Fish
Stonefly
Mayfly

Fish
Shrimps
Caddisfly

Tubificid worms
Red chironomids
Rat-tailed maggots

Water louse
Snails

Dissolved oxygen (% saturation)

100

80

60

40

20

Clean water | Deaeration | Zone of critical oxygen deficit | Recovery | Clean water

Distance downstream from discharge point ⟶

Figure 2.4
**This diagram shows the effects on the composition of the aquatic
community following discharge of organic waste.**

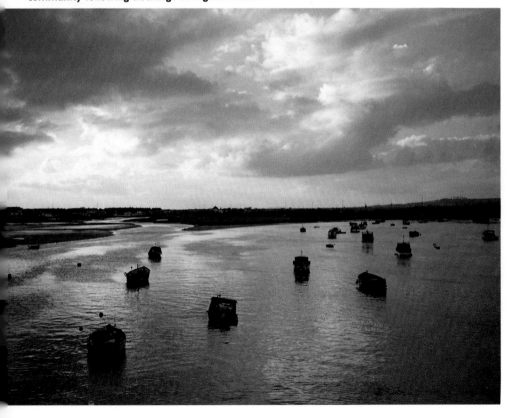

**Estuaries are critical
breeding areas for
many aquatic
organisms, but are
susceptible to pollution
from river and sea
discharges.**

raised or lowered by the tide. The best indicator of water quality in estuaries are the biota. In the freshwater zone the organisms are predominantly those natural to the freshwater environment; the seawater zone contains marine organisms; and the transitional or 'inter-haline' zone contains a large diversity of both sea- and freshwater species. Estuaries are areas of high biotic activity and are often critical breeding areas for many aquatic organisms. Because estuaries are usually bordered by low lying land, there can be considerable freshwater discharge into them, but in a dry summer it can also take several months for water to travel from the tidal limit to the sea, with serious implications for bathers since any sewage pollution will become concentrated.

Seas and oceans

Oceans are the ultimate sinks of the products of land erosion and of the impurities in rainwater. They are also the ultimate destination for most of the end-products of man-made pollution of the air and water. Water discharged to the sea does not usually contain much readily degradable organic matter; this has been largely broken down already to simple compounds in rivers and estuaries. However, seas and oceans are massive sources of primary production of organic matter by phytoplankton, the starting point of all natural aquatic food chains. The degree to which ocean waters are contaminated by toxic substances is very low. There are very small traces of heavy metals, derived mainly from land run-off. Some species of marine plankton do contain naturally produced organic toxins which are either harmful to fish or to humans consuming the fish.

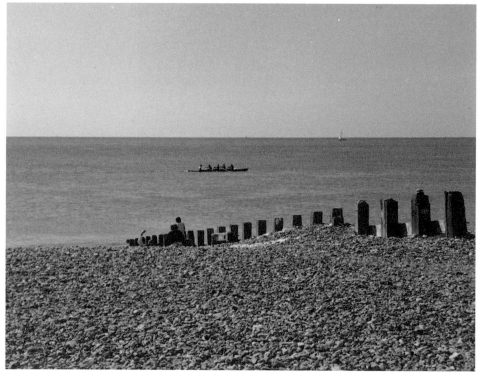

Oceans are often the final destination for environmental pollution.

Enclosed sea basins in which there is little circulation to disperse pollutants are becoming increasingly stressed because of discharges of industrial effluent and sewage. Parts of the Mediterranean are biologically dead, and areas within both the North and Baltic Seas contain fish and mammals suffering from diseases caused by discharge of sludge and toxic materials.

SOURCES OF WATER POLLUTION

In some parts of the country the water tastes so unpleasant that there is clear public concern about its quality. But most of the 700 or so known chemical contaminants are not detectable to the eye, the nose or the taste buds. Many of the chemicals in drinking water are harmless; others are demonstrably harmful; for the majority there is no clear proof one way or another. One of the key difficulties faced by scientists in assessing the potential health risks arises from what is popularly called 'the cocktail effect'. This problem can be illustrated by reference to pesticide residues in food.

According to the Government's Steering Group on Food Surveillance, 'At present toxicological interpretation is particularly difficult where residues of more than one pesticide are found in the same [food] sample'[23]. A similar point has been made by WHO, about mixtures of certain pesticides in drinking water: 'The problem of exposure to any mixture of two or more of the herbicides . . . cannot be handled in isolation. . . . Drinking water may contain chemical residues of different types, including pesticides, other environmental contaminants, or micropollutants, many of which may as yet be unidentified. In addition, people are exposed to chemical substances by many other routes, which may give rise to possible interactions. The complexity of the problem precludes simple answers'[49].

WHO recommend that 'the possible toxicological implications of such contamination should be assessed on a case-by-case basis . . . all available information on the toxicological properties of the individual substances must be collected in order to assess the hazard of each substance'[49].

Water pollution occurs in several ways:

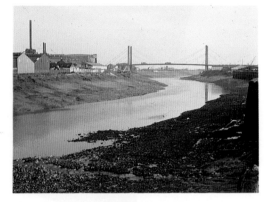
River life may be destroyed by discharges from factories and power stations.

1 *Physical* pollution takes place when solid debris is put into streams, smothering life on the stream-bed, or when relatively hot water from factories and power stations is discharged into a river. The rise in temperature of the river water lowers the available, dissolved oxygen which supports life critical for the self-purification processes taking place in the river.
2 *Biological* pollution arises when living things are added to water; for example, human disease-causing organisms of faecal origin in sewage effluent. Discharges of biodegradable, organic chemicals may also upset the natural balance of organisms in a stream, promote excessive growth and lower oxygen levels to critical levels.
3 *Chemical* pollution is the addition of chemical contaminants to water. The major cause is discharge of wastewater from urban areas. Other important sources are spillages of oil and industrial chemicals, disposal of sludges to the sea,

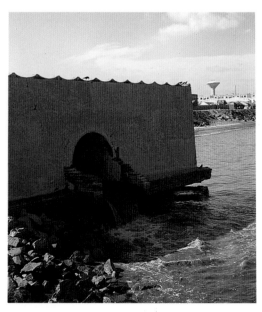
Sewers like this, discharge effluent directly into the sea.

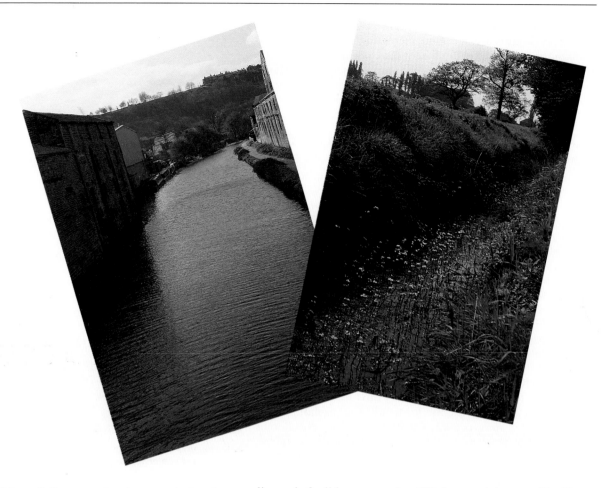

Water pollution occurs in urban or agricultural areas.

disposal of solid wastes on landfill sites, and the use of fertilizers and pesticides in agriculture.

A realistic definition of water pollution, offered by the Royal Society of Chemistry, is: 'Any man-made alteration of the chemical, physical or biological quality of a water which results in an unacceptable depreciation of the utility or environmental value of the water'[48].

PESTICIDES IN WATER

Pesticides may enter water supplies from several sources. These include careless overspraying of water courses, drains or standing water; run-off from sprayed or treated areas; careless disposal of containers; the illegal disposal of waste pesticides in farm soakaways; washing down of contaminated equipment; spills; and leaching from soil in treated areas. On occasions pesticides, particularly pyrethroids, are deliberately added to water supplies to control infestations of asellus and water shrimps in water mains. The doses of pyrethroids are very small (less than 0.03 mg l^{-1}) and closely controlled, but can harm aquarium fish and are drunk by the public. The risk to humans is very low since the levels of dosing are also very low, added to which are the benefits to water companies of having a greatly reduced number of complaints of finding asellus and water shrimps in tap water. Water companies are also replacing chemical dosing by physical cleaning using foam swabs and air scouring.

A considerable number of common pesticides have been detected in water supplies as a result of routine monitoring. In evidence to the Agriculture Committee on the Effects of Pesticides on Human Health[2] the Department of the Environment informed the committee that triazines (herbicides), particularly atrazine, have been detected in many supplies derived from both surface and ground-water sources. Phenoxyalkanoic acid compounds (herbicides), particularly mecocrop and MCPA but also 2,4-D and MCPB, have been detected in surface- and ground-water derived supplies in intensive and arable agricultural areas. Other pesticides, such as the persistent organochlorine compounds, have been detected occasionally. The Anglian Water Authority provided evidence of contamination of both surface and ground-water. The principal pesticides detected in surface water were mecocrop, atrazine, simazine, dimethoate and lindane, which were each found regularly at the great majority of monitoring sites. Dimethoate, mecocrop, and atrazine were also found at 10% of the ground-water monitoring sites, but at levels within WHO limits.

As with nitrate, there is particular concern in some quarters about the contamination of ground-water by persistent pesticides. While some pesticides degrade quickly in water by hydrolysis – which is a reaction of the pesticide and water itself – others are not degraded in this way and can contaminate ground-water: one example is atrazine. If the ground-water is then pumped up for drinking purposes, there is the possibility of a low level of pesticide exposure to the population. There are also concerns that disinfection of the water with chlorine may convert pesticides into different chemicals with different toxicological properties, and that this would complicate any assessment of the possible effects of pesticide residues in drinking water. However, these are largely theoretical, because the addition of chloride to the water tends to hasten the degradation of pesticides. In fact, this process is used in manufacturing to clean up effluents from manufacturing plants.

Levels of pesticides in drinking water are regulated by a European Community Directive on quality of water intended for human consumption (80/778/EEC). The directive came into force in July 1985 and sets the Maximum Admissible Concentration (MAC) for any single pesticide at 0.1 μg l^{-1} (that is, one part per ten billion) and total pesticides at 0.5 μg l^{-1}. In June 1987 Friends of the Earth (FoE) wrote to all water suppliers in England and Wales requesting information about compliance with the MAC for pesticides (Figure 2.5). The evidence collected[50] suggested that the MAC for single pesticides was exceeded in 298 water sources/supplies, and breaches of the MAC for total pesticides were recorded on 76 occasions. The detected breaches were all in England, specifically in the Anglian, North West, Severn-Trent, Thames, Wessex and Yorkshire Regions. The absence of reported breaches from elsewhere in England, and in Wales, may reflect inadequate investigations in these areas. Sixteen pesticides (active ingredients) were each detected at levels above the MAC for a single pesticide. The most commonly detected were atrazine and simazine which were regularly measured above

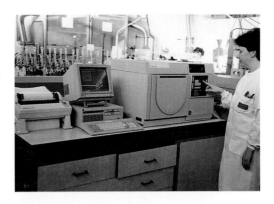

Some of the chemicals detected in drinking water are harmless, but for many there is no clear proof of long-term safety.

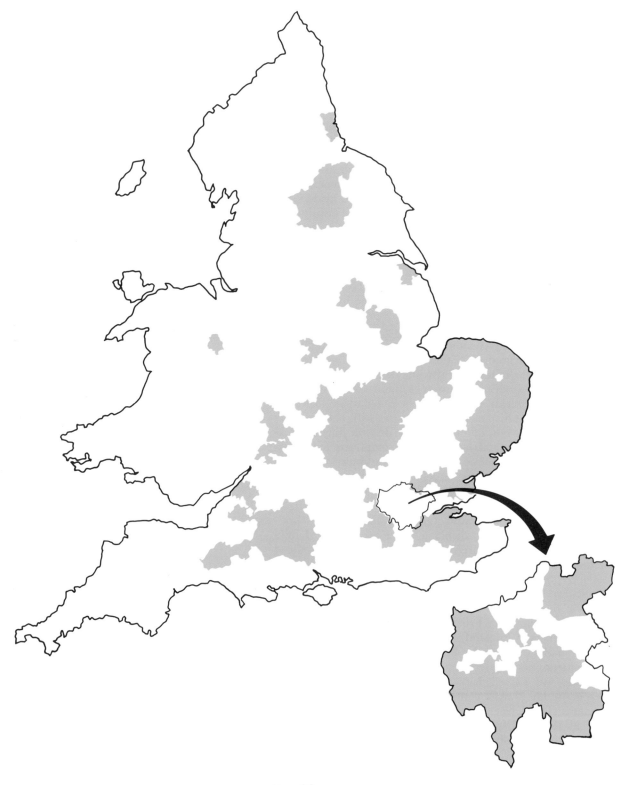

Figure 2.5
A 1987 survey by Friends of the Earth revealed that many drinking water supplies in the UK exceeded the permissable level of pesticides.

the MAC throughout much of the Anglian, Wessex, Severn-Trent and Thames regions. They are widely used as 'total weedkillers' by British Rail, local councils and industry.

On 1 September 1989, the Water Supply (Water Quality) Regulations 1989 came into force in England and Wales reinforcing EC regulations; these must be complied with by water companies in meeting the MACs.

However, the FoE report states that their results significantly understated the scale of the problem. They claim that the Government's current advice ensures that most water suppliers do not test drinking water frequently for low levels of many pesticides, let alone the other toxic components of pesticide formulations or their breakdown products. The ability of water suppliers to assess compliance with the MACs for pesticides in drinking water is currently undermined by a shortage of suitable analytical techniques, and the high cost of using those techniques that are available. Furthermore, few water suppliers sample surface water sources often enough to assess seasonal variations in pesticide levels. The situation is compounded by a paucity of accurate data about the extent of water pollution by pesticides, the possible health risks and potentially unreliable safety tests, particularly for older pesticides. This inadequacy of existing data has been recognized by several other bodies, including the 1979 Royal Commission on Environmental Pollution[3] and the 1987 Agriculture Committee[2].

When pesticides are tested for their animal and ecological toxicity they are not tested in their pure form. The material used is that which contains the impurities present in the manufacturing process. Thus safety testing is relevant to human exposure. It is necessary to take into account the whole body intake of pesticides via food and air, as well as the small amount that may be drunk. WHO has adopted this philosophy in compiling its *Guidelines for Drinking Water Quality*.

In March 1989 the Government announced a programme for the routine review of the safety of over 100 older pesticides. Priority will be given to 'those active ingredients which have been approved the longest and are most widely used.' The Government says that the pesticides are those where 'no particular concern exists but where the age of the supporting data suggests re-evaluation to modern-day standards would be appropriate'. In other words, the Government cannot guarantee that a large number of widely used pesticides are safe by today's standards.

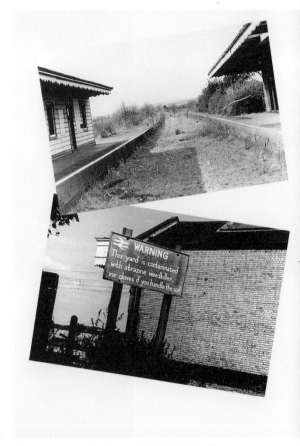

Atrazine contamination of this British Rail site clearly shows the potency and long-term effects of this total weedkiller.

OTHER SOURCES OF WATER CONTAMINATION

Wastewater and Water Pollution

Wastewater originates from domestic use and from industry. Run-off from concreted or built-on land may end up directly in the drainage system rather than in ground-water. Some 96% of the water used in UK households becomes wastewater, or domestic sewage. The total volume of this sewage in the UK amounts to 14 million cubic metres (3100 million gallons) per day[51]. Nearly all households in the UK discharge their drainage to public sewers and thence to sewage treatment works, which

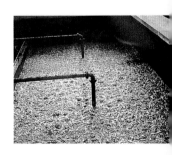

Almost all the water used in UK households is discharged into sewers and treated at a sewage treatment plant.

Drainge water discharged onto a beach.

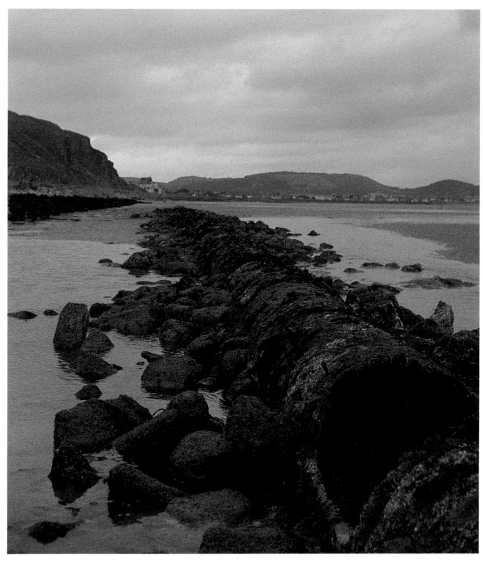

in turn discharge to rivers or coastal waters. A few sewage works discharge their effluent to underground rocks, and some rural households have their own septic tanks. These drain liquid wastes into the ground, but need to be desludged periodically by tanker to control solid deposits.

Industrial wastewater also drains into public sewers or even directly into rivers. It may or may not be treated at sewage works, but inevitably ends up in our streams and rivers. The total daily production of industrial wastewater in England and Wales amounts to some 12 million cubic metres a day. Agricultural wastewaters are mainly disposed of by being returned to the land, sometimes after storage and treatment. Streams, rivers and coastal waters are therefore the main recipients of treated (and sometimes not so treated) wastewater. At present, there is no other economically practicable way of disposal, so our attention needs to focus on the best way of ensuring that the chemicals that we discharge into our aquatic environment cause the minimum level of damage both to our environment and to our health.

Chemicals in water

The wastewater directed into our rivers contains a variety of pollutants. Those generated by the paper industry (non-degradable organic and chlorine based substances), the metal-working industry (dissolved and particulate compounds of heavy metals, chromium, nickel, zinc, cadmium, and lead, as well as iron and titanium oxides) and the petrochemical industry (phenols and mineral oils) are particularly damaging to rivers, lakes and canals. Slaughterhouses, breweries, tanneries, textile works and many other processes make their own contributions.

Modern processing methods, legislation and research and development programmes have all helped to reduce water pollution. But despite these efforts water reserves are still at considerable risk of pollution. Non-degradable industrial chemicals such as organohalogen compounds (for example, chloroform, trichloroethylene, carbon tetrachloride, and DDT), polycyclic aromatic hydrocarbons, pesticides, and polychlorinated biphenyls (PCBs) have not only been detected in sewage but also in rainwater, surface water, ground-water, seawater and in drinking water supplies.

Water in an aquifer is replaced very slowly and any toxic chemicals can contaminate groundwater supplies for many years to come.

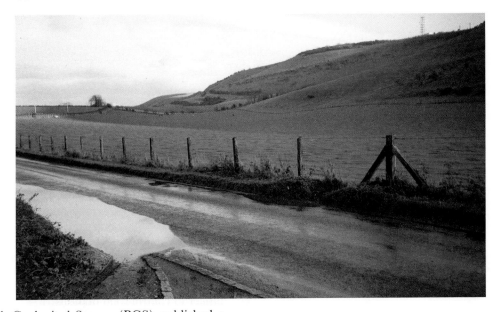

In 1987 the British Geological Survey (BGS) published a study of *The Pollution Threat from Agricultural Pesticides and Solvents*[52]. The report concluded that the assumption that chemicals decay quickly in soil or simply evaporate is no longer valid. Although some compounds are rapidly hydrolysed in water, others break down very slowly and can percolate swiftly into aquifers, particularly through sandy soils and chalk. The most serious problems occur when chemicals penetrate ground-water (Figure 2.6). A river is constantly renewing itself: water flows out to sea and is replaced by water coming down off the hills. The whole river is permanently being flushed out. But once chemicals have contaminated ground-water supplies, pollution can affect the supply for decades before it is reduced to 'safe' levels[53].

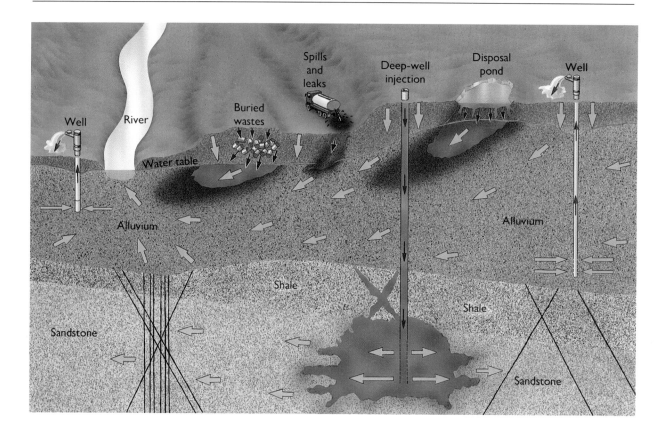

Figure 2.6
Pollutants which are dumped into rivers, buried in landfill sites, or placed in deep wells may eventually find their way into groundwater supplies.

Among problem pesticides, 'the most widespread threat is likely to be associated with certain herbicides, especially the carboxyacid and phenylurea groups, which are very widely and regularly applied for weed control in cereal production on the permeable soils of aquifer outcrops. . . . Some compounds are highly toxic at very low concentrations close to detection limits and therefore highly sophisticated analytical procedures are required.'

The BGS report takes a similar view of solvents, reporting that 'the common chlorinated organic solvents are potentially very serious and most insidious ground-water pollutants . . . even a spill of a few litres in volume could, in theory, contaminate many millions of litres of ground-water'[52]. Accidental discharges of even less than 1 litre of some chlorinated solvents could kill all the working bacteria in a sewage treatment works.

In response to the concern evident in the BGS report and from many other sources, the Government is now taking action to improve the quality of drinking water. The Department of the Environment recently circulated a consultation paper on control of dangerous substances in water, which proposed a selection scheme to identify a limited range of the most dangerous substances in water (the 'Red List') and recommended measures to reduce inputs of these substances from different sources. The Red List is drawn from EC Directive 76/464 on dangerous substances in water, which included a 'List 1' of 129 substances, selected on the basis of their toxicity, persistence, and potential for bioaccumulation: 23 substances have been identified as requiring stricter controls when discharged into

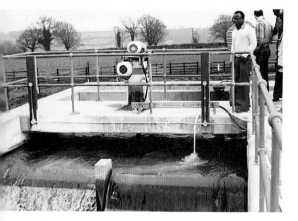

Water purification.

rivers, estuaries and sewers. The list includes mercury, cadmium, polychlorinated biphenyls and 16 pesticides: DDT, PCP, HCB, aldrin, dieldrin, endrin, triorganotin compounds, dichlorvos, azinphosmethyl, fenitrothion, malathion, endosulfan, atrazine, and simazine. A further list of 23 'priority candidates' for inclusion in the Red List is appended and ten of these are pesticides. In publishing the list, Britain has agreed to measures that will halve discharges of these especially toxic compounds, which persist in water and accumulate in living organisms. Under the proposed new controls, companies will have to reduce discharges by applying the best available techniques not entailing excessive cost, but in practice, the treatment technology will only reach the minimum levels required by law (Figure 2.7).

Figure 2.7
Dangerous substances found in domestic water supplies often come from particular industries.

	Fertiliser Industry	Pesticide Industry	Petroleum Refining	Petrochemical Industry	Chemical Industry	Pulp/paper Industry	Metal/metal Plating	Textile Industry	Iron/steel Industry
Chlorinated Organic Compounds	✓	✓		✓	✓	✓	✓	✓	
Minerals & Oils	✓		✓	✓	✓	✓	✓	✓	✓
Phenols			✓	✓	✓	✓	✓		✓
Nitrogen	✓		✓	✓	✓	✓	✓	✓	✓
Phosphorus	✓	✓			✓	✓		✓	
Mercury	✓	✓		✓	✓	✓	✓		✓
Lead	✓			✓	✓		✓		✓
Cadmium	✓				✓		✓		✓

Veterinary Drugs

Some public concern has focused on residues of veterinary drugs in meat. Intakes are monitored by the Steering Group on Food Surveillance, whose 1988 report *Anabolic, Anthelminthic and Antimicrobial Agents*[54] covered 10 years of sampling. For example, national surveys of sulphonamide residues in kidney samples, particularly pig kidney, found that 13% contained residues in excess of the acceptable level of sulphadimidine, leading to action by MAFF in 1986 which in turn has led to a reduction in residues. Concern over the use of sulphonamide relates to both resistance in the target organisms, and possible sensitization and allergic reactions in man. There has been

High levels of sulphonamide residues in pig kidneys, prompted government action in 1986 which successfully led to a reduction in residues.

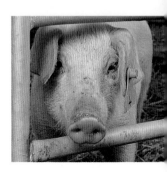

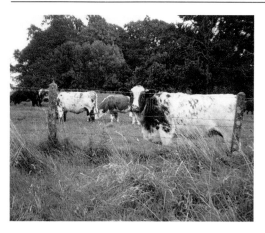

The use of growth promoting hormones and anabolic steroids in livestock was banned by the EC in 1988.

Most of the world's domestic and hazardous wastes are disposed of in landfills.

discussion about the adverse effects on human health of hormones and anabolic steroids which may be given to animals to promote rapid weight gain. In 1980 children in Milan experienced premature sexual maturing, which was blamed on consumption of veal which had been treated with a female sex hormone from the stilbene group. Although the connection was not proved, stilbenes were banned by international agreement in 1981. In 1988 the EC banned the use of both growth promoting hormones and anabolic steroids in livestock[55], although the products have been approved by licensing authorities in parts of the developed world, and have been passed also by the WHO and the UN Food and Agriculture Association via the Codex Alimentarius.

Industrial Pollutants

More than 90% of the world's domestic and hazardous wastes are disposed of in landfills[47]. At its most primitive, landfilling consists of no more than tipping waste into a hole in the ground, although modern landfill sites are specially engineered, with waste being tipped into special, clay-lined, impervious cells. Unlined 'dilute and disperse' sites can allow toxic chemicals to pollute ground-water, even though the theory behind them is that natural chemical and biological processes will render the waste harmless as it seeps through the underlying soil. Fears about 'dilute and disperse' pollution have led several countries to limit landfilling to 'containment' sites. These sites are lined with impermeable material such as clay or plastic, or built over impermeable soil. However, heavy rain can cause the sites to overflow and some of the chemicals, particularly industrial

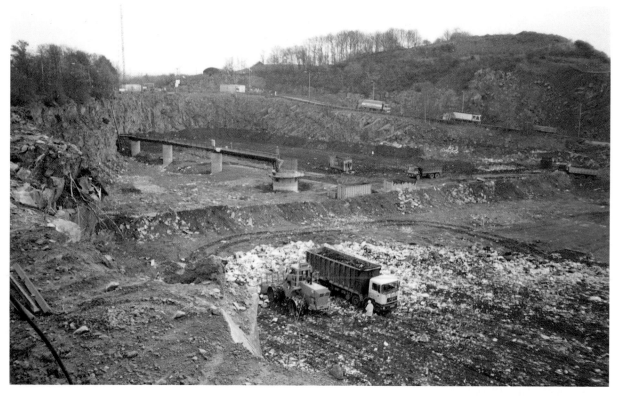

solvents, can eventually penetrate the lining. The liquid drain-ing from a waste dump (the 'leachate') may contain a wide range of concentrated pollutants such as heavy metals, solvents, ammonia, phenols and cyanides. These pollutants are some-times trapped in drains around the site and then pumped back on top of the site. Very little is known of how leacheates may react during their movement through the unsaturated zone to the water table.

Toxic waste disposal is a growth industry. This toxic waste is not only the product of British industry: in 1981 4000 tonnes of toxic or 'special' waste were imported. By 1987 it was up to 53 000 tonnes (and more was probably imported illegally)[45]. This trade came to public attention in the summer of 1988 when a ship called the *Karin B* attempted to land 2000 tonnes of toxic waste in the UK.

Many waste products are disposed of in landfill sites, as described above. Other waste is pumped directly into rivers or into water authority sewers. Twelve million cubic metres of industrial wastewater are discharged into the water system every day. Inevitably there is pollution. The Control of Pollu-tion Act 1974 made factories subject to discharge consents agreed with the local water authority. This legal duty now comes under the Water Act 1989, and discharge consents are now agreed with the National Rivers Authority (NRA), and with the River Purification Boards in Scotland. Despite this there have been many infringements. In 1988 there were 23 000 reported pollution incidents in Britain, double the figure for 1982, and industry was responsible for 37% of them[53]. During the past few decades it has been argued that criminal law is too blunt an instrument for pollution control. What has been proposed is a system of charges or taxes calculated according to the damage that results from the quantity and quality of the discharge: the 'polluter pay' principle.

A number of recent incidents have highlighted the problems of water contamination by industrial chemicals. A 1984 public enquiry into ground-water pollution in Norwich identified the source as the nearby May and Baker chemical factory. Under-ground water was found to be contaminated with bromide, sulphate, benzene, toluene and other chemicals. Despite the efforts of the company and frequent inspections by the water authority, it was clear that a number of spillages and con-taminations had occurred. In 1988 in Andover, Southern Water found that a spillage of over 450 litres of chlorinated solvents had contaminated a borehole. These solvents are used in paper making, metal plating and electrical engineering, as well as in dry cleaning. The chemicals can leak from storage tanks and seep down into the ground-water, sometimes ending up thou-sands of metres away. In another incident involving industrial solvents, a routine sample of water taken in Suffolk in 1981 revealed the presence of solvents in an aquifer supplying 40 000 people. The source of the pollution was traced to the US Air Force base at RAF Mildenhall, and a major public supply borehole had to be closed.

In 1989 an oil pipeline under the River Mersey burst owing to poor maintenance and the new NRA prosecuted the pipeline owner, Shell, who were fined £1 million. The *Exxon Valdez* incident in Alaska in 1989 also illustrates the extremely damaging effects of oil pollution. Even small spills cause monolayers of oil on the surface, which reduce the transfer of oxygen into the water.

Phosphates and Detergents

During the 1950s the introduction of synthetic washing powders had a dramatic effect on many of Britain's rivers. Residues of detergent, not destroyed by the normal sewage treatment process caused widespread visible pollution, including large, mobile aggregates of bubbles known as 'swans'[56]. Oxygen levels were reduced by these residues, which were also toxic to fish, and sewage works which inject oxygen into sewage suffered because these materials interfered with purification processes and the works were covered with foam. Since then voluntary agreements between the Government and detergent manufacturers have led to a move to 'softer', more biodegradable detergents for domestic use, although 'hard' detergents are still used in industry. In the main this agreement has been successful, although there has been some pollution of rivers receiving hard, detergent effluent from the textile industry.

A problem that still exists arises from the use of phosphates as water softeners in synthetic detergents. Phosphates from detergents make up about half the phosphate content of domestic sewage, the rest coming from natural human wastes. Fertiliser phosphate, another source of phosphate, is strongly absorbed by soil particles and carried off only by erosion, and is therefore a smaller source than animal excreta. In the early 1960s it was noticed that numerous lakes and reservoirs, particularly in industrialised countries, seemed to be undergoing a process of 'accelerated eutrophication.'

Water pollution by detergents can cause the formation of large mobile aggregates of bubbles known as "swans".

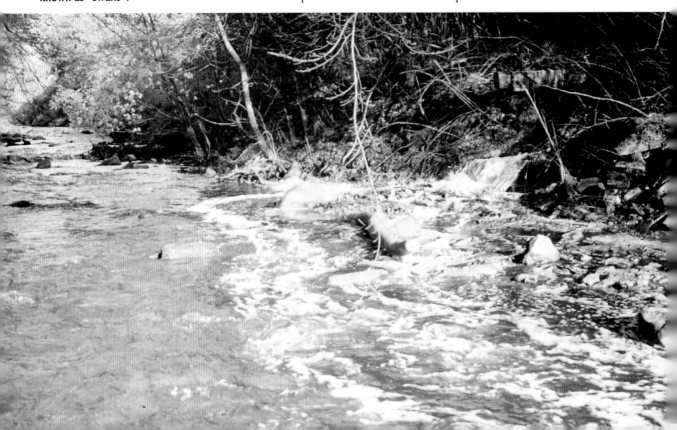

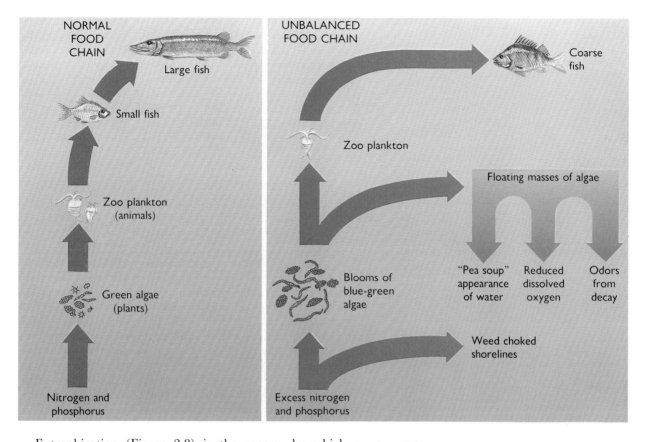

Eutrophication (Figure 2.8) is the process by which a
stream or lake becomes increasingly richer in plant nutrients,
usually nitrates and phosphates. Typically there is then heavy
growth of aquatic plants and mats of algae, and there is
deoxygenation of the water, which becomes foul smelling and
virtually lifeless. Accelerated eutrophication has been caused
largely by excessive nutrient enrichment from human activities.
The main nutrient sources are municipal and industrial wastewaters, and agricultural and urban run-offs. These contribute
many tonnes of nitrates and phosphates to the freshwater and
marine environments every year[48]. A study by the Organisation
for Economic Co-operation and Development (OECD) in
1982[57] collected data on eutrophication from 150 lakes, ranging
from ponds to the North American Great Lakes. The contributions made by nitrates, phosphates and other factors were
statistically evaluated and, almost without exception, phosphorus was found to be the factor determining the development
of eutrophication. In the UK there are some bodies of water (the
Broads, Loch Leven and Lough Neagh) which have had eutrophication problems. In the case of Lough Neagh the problem
was solved by removing phosphate at the ten sewage works
around the Lough. Similarly, in the Norfolk Broads, where
there is serious phosphate pollution, a plant has been built to
remove phosphates from sewage before it is discharged into
local rivers. Algae in lakes in the UK is not normally a problem
unless long periods of fine, sunny and calm weather allows a
warm layer of water to stabilize at the surface. Algae can then

Figure 2.8
**The normal aquatic food chain is altered when a
body of water becomes algae-choked due to
eutrophication.**

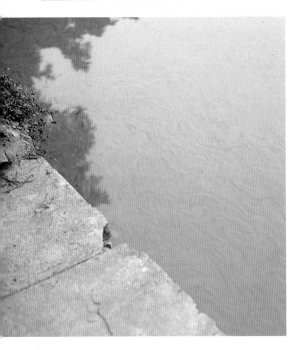

Toxin-producing blue-green algae cause skin irritation and can be fatal to dogs and sheep.

thrive, and some toxin-producing blue–green algae will cause skin irritation and even kill dogs, sheep and fish. This happened in Rutland Water reservoir in the East Midlands during the summer of 1989. Footpaths around the lakes were closed and water recreation activities were stopped for several months.

In the early 1980s there were attempts to introduce alternatives to phosphates as water softeners. Unfortunately some of the substitutes have proved to be more hazardous than the phosphates they were intended to replace. These include NTA (nitrilo-tri-acetic acid) and EDTA (ethylene diamino-tetra-acetic acid). NTA is now banned in the USA because it combines with heavy metals, such as lead and mercury, and makes them even more difficult to remove from the water supply by ordinary treatment processes.

Aluminium

Every year 100 000 tonnes of aluminium sulphate are deliberately added to the water supply in some treatment works by the water companies. This is to help a process called flocculation which causes fine, suspended material to coagulate and sink to the bottom of conical storage tanks. Lime slurry is often added with the aluminium sulphate and the two react together to form tiny particles of aluminium hydroxide, which attract each other and remain in suspension balanced by the upward flow of water in the tanks. The particles attract other fine particles to them. The water passing through the blanket of flocculating aluminium hydroxide is skimmed off the top of the tanks and is then sand filtered to remove any clumps of insoluble material which may also have been washed over the top. This clean, sparkling water is then disinfected by chlorine before leaving the treatment works; but if the aluminium dosing is not closely controlled, there is a chance that some aluminium may be introduced into the supply by the treatment.

The directive from the European Commission on drinking water specifies a limit on aluminium in tap water of 0.2 parts per million. Many areas of Britain may not meet this specification, in particular those areas where there is acid rain. Acid rain falling on parts of Europe can dissolve aluminium from rocks, which may not be removed by waterworks treatment.

In July 1988 there was a serious water pollution incident at the Lowermoor water treatment works in Cornwall when a 20 tonne load of 8% solution of aluminium sulphate was accidentally dumped in the water supply. Following the incident many of the residents of Camelford complained of experiencing mouth ulcers, blisters, sore throats, irritation of the skin, scalp rashes and bleached hair. There were also complaints of lassitude, malaise and diarrhoea. These symptoms may have been caused by copper poisoning as a result of acid water attacking the copper scale of hot water systems[58]. A panel of enquiry, chaired by Dame Barbara Clayton of Southampton University, criticised the South West Water Authority for giving contradictory, confusing and inappropriate advice which, coupled with alarmist reports in the media, served only to increase anxiety. It was this anxiety, concluded the report, and not the toxic effects of the chemical, which caused most of the symptoms recorded in Camelford[58].

It may be some years before the possible long-term health effects of the Lowermoor incident become apparent (although there is no on-going survey taking place that could identify those effects). There is already growing evidence that a high aluminium content in drinking water appears to contribute to bone disease. There is tentative evidence that aluminium could be at least partially responsible for Alzheimer's disease. It has been known for some time that patients using high aluminium water for kidney dialysis could suffer from dementia – the so-called 'dialysis dementia'[55]. Now attention is focusing on the role of aluminium in dementia in the elderly[59]. In addition to ingesting aluminium in drinking water, elderly people may also be taking in large amounts of active aluminium in medicines such as antacids and aspirin. They may have difficulty also in secreting excess aluminium because their kidneys are functioning less well.

The water supply companies are reducing and controlling the amounts of aluminium flocculants in water treatment and in some cases are using other coagulants such as iron salts. The UK prescribed concentration is set at 0.2 mg l^{-1} (parts per million).

Lead

Lead is probably the best documented of all known poisons. Even the Roman architect Vitruvius was aware of the dangers of lead pipes. Lead reaches us in several ways. Lead in petrol has been a major public issue in recent years. Lead in paint, particularly the older high-lead varieties, has caused a number of fatalities and in the USA there are laws restricting the amount of lead in paint to 600 parts per million. In the UK there is no such law, although paints containing large quantities must be labelled. Lead residues are also found in food, originating from airborne lead and lead solders in food cans. Another significant source is lead plumbing. Most houses built before 1964 have some lead pipework, but this was banned from use in domestic plumbing systems in that year. Those most at risk are people who live in older houses in acidic water areas, including most of Scotland, the North of England, Wales and the West Country. Cities affected include Glasgow, Edinburgh, Birmingham, Manchester, Liverpool and Hull (Figure 2.9). A survey carried out in 1975–76 showed that 7% of water samples taken from taps in England had levels of lead exceeding the EC safety limit of 100 µg l^{-1}. In Scotland the corresponding figure was 34%[47]. Since then the EC has recognized that, although 100 µg l^{-1} remains the upper limit for a safe level of lead in drinking water, a lower figure of 50 µg l^{-1} should be used as the maximum acceptable lead level in a 'flushed' sample, that is one where the water has been allowed to run before testing.

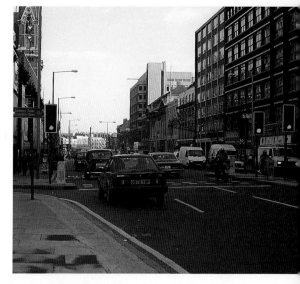

Lead may be released into the environment from vehicle exhaust.

The Department of the Environment's Pollution Paper on *Lead in the Environment*[60] noted that the lead content of the public water supply in the UK is well below even the lower limit prescribed by the European Community. It is in the distribution system – usually the domestic plumbing system – that amounts of more than trace lead can get into the supply. The major factor governing the amount of lead in the water is the presence of soft, acid water; but pipe length and condition, the

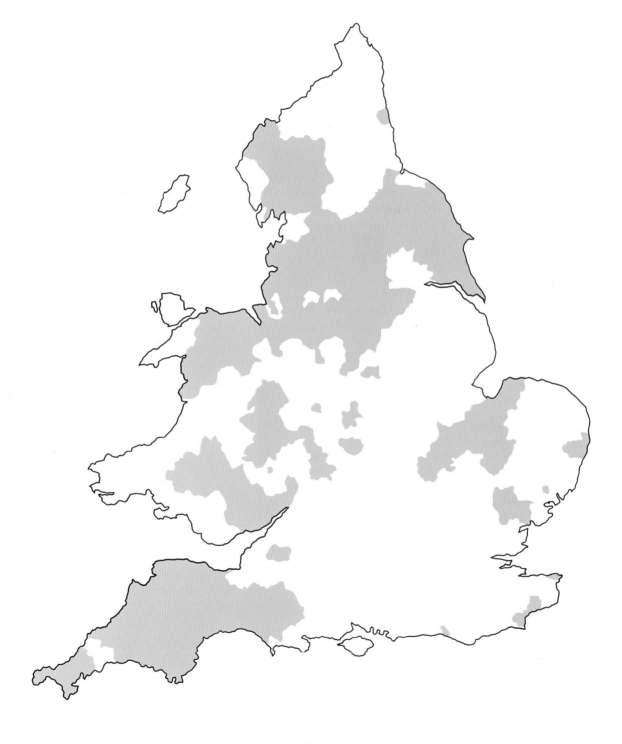

Figure 2.9
**A 1987 survey by Friends of the Earth revealed that in parts of the
country the level of lead in drinking water exceeded the EC limit.**

time the water has stood in the pipe or tank and the rate at which the water flows through the system all make their contribution.

The 1989 Water Act has now prescribed 50 µg l^{-1} (0.05 mg l^{-1}) as the maximum permissible lead concentration in any tap sample whether the system has been flushed or not. The recently published government report on *Lead in Food*[61] noted that results from diet studies and from unpublished data on blood lead levels for people exposed to about 50 µg l^{-1} lead in water indicate that for adults average water lead concentrations should not exceed about 30 µg l^{-1}. For bottle-fed infants the average lead concentrations should not exceed 10–15 µg l^{-1}. Treatment processes are being introduced in areas of risk, which include addition of calcium and bicarbonates to make the water alkaline and therefore less corrosive to the metal in the pipes, but the problem of corrosion is not simply solved by water treatment and will be costly to rectify totally. Many cases of lead poisoning are due entirely to household plumbing. Mains water may have a very low lead content but could dissolve lead in the service pipe connecting a house to the mains. Lead service pipes could be replaced by plastic ones, but the consumer will inevitably have to pay.

Lead, once released to the environment, remains 'available' for a long time compared with many other chemicals. Because of its lengthy persistence and potential toxicity to a very wide range of organisms it is a pollutant of particular significance. The effects of acute lead poisoning are clear enough: stomach pains, headaches, tremor, irritability and, in severe cases, coma and death. In the long term, lead is known to affect the brain and nerves at low concentrations. Many authorities now accept that levels of lead commonly found in the blood of urban children has a significant effect on their mental development and functioning, so by reducing the levels of lead in drinking water the total amount of lead ingested can be lowered. While the introduction of lead-free petrol will go some way towards the reduction of lead in the atmosphere, it is still necessary to reduce particulate lead in the environment which can be respired or absorbed.

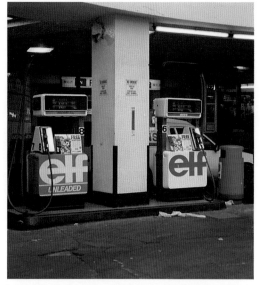

Lead-free fuel makes a valuable contribution to lowering the amount of lead in the environment.

Nitrate

Nitrate is the end product of the decay of nitrogenous material such as nitrogen fertilizers, animal excreta and dead plants and animals. Nitrate levels in ground-water and surface water in most of the UK have been rising steadily over the past few decades (Figure 2.10).

The amount of nitrate in surface water fluctuates with the seasons, influencing algae and plant growth rates which can degrade stream and lake water quality. Increased discharges of sewage in lowland rivers also increases the level of nitrate. Farming practices since 1940 have contributed to rising levels of nitrate infiltrating ground-water. It will take years before controls implemented on discharges of sewage and on farming practice will be reflected in a fall in the levels of nitrate in the deeper aquifers.

Bottle-fed infants especially those under 9 months of age are at risk if the nitrate value is at or above 50 mg l^{-1} as NO_3 in the

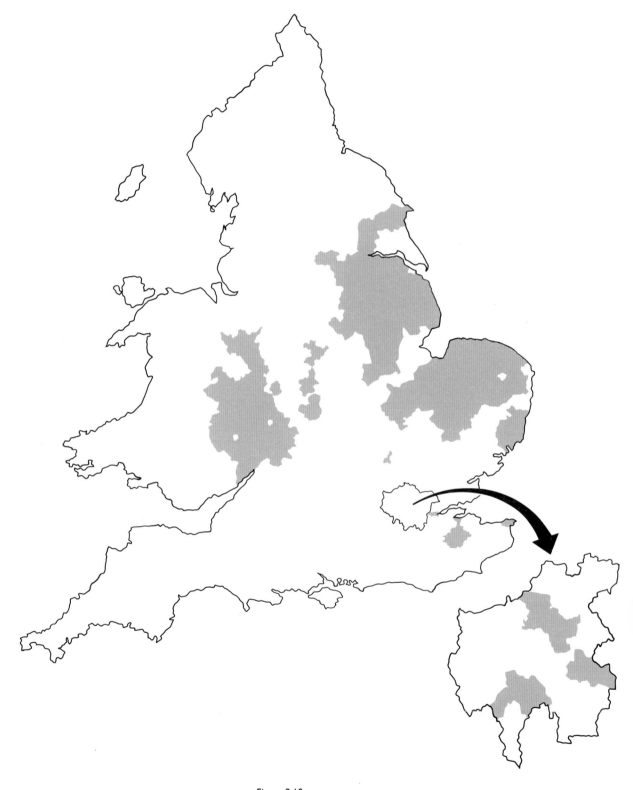

Figure 2.10
**A 1987 survey of Friends of the Earth revealed that a number of
drinking water supplies throughout the country contained nitrate in
excess of the EC limit.**

water used for feed preparation. Nitrate in the water can be converted to nitrites in infants' stomachs which, when absorbed through the digestive system, react with blood to form methaemoglobin. Methaemoglobin prevents oxygen being absorbed by the blood circulating in the lungs, causing cyanosis, or blue baby syndrome. In the UK the risk is well identified, and there have been no cases of high nitrate in water causing any deaths since 1948. Evidence that high nitrate in water may cause cancer in adults is inconclusive[62].

It has been estimated that up to £15 million per year may be needed to reduce nitrate in UK water supplies to EC limits. Treatment processes for nitrate removal using ion exchange denitrification plants have been installed by two water companies in the UK.

Pathogens

Pathogens are disease-causing organisms. Water polluted by faeces and sewage may contain many different pathogens, among which are those causing cholera, typhoid, diarrhoea and dysentery. Biological pathogens include cryptosporidium and amoebae. Bacteriological pathogens are responsible for cholera and typhoid, while hepatitis, polio and certain types of diarrhoea are caused by viruses which can be transmitted in water. Pathogen-caused diseases usually appear very quickly after infection and their severity varies from mild gastroenteric upsets to severe and fatal illnesses of epidemic proportions depending on the age, nutritional status and general health of the population affected and the infective dose (reproducing bacteria are capable of doubling their numbers every 20 minutes).

In public health terms, it is the microbiological quality of drinking water that is of the greatest importance. In Europe and North America, rigorous, continual monitoring takes place to detect any organisms indicative of faecal pollution in drinking water supplies. Such microbiological quality control is lacking in other parts of the world, so that in the developing countries over 30000 children die each day from diseases triggered by polluted water and poor sanitation.

Cryptosporidiosis occurred in the Oxford and Swindon areas during 1989, indicating that water companies must be continually vigilant in monitoring water supplies for pathogens. The illness is usually mild with diarrhoea, abdominal cramps and sometimes fever that resolves in 1–3 weeks. It can affect people of any age but is most common in children between the ages of 1 and 5 years. According to the interim report by the Department of the Environment Group of Experts issued in July 1989: 'In patients with AIDS and others whose resistance to infection is impaired, it (cryptosporidiosis) is much more serious and may lead to severe and lasting disability.'

WATER PURIFICATION

Most water requires treatment before it is suitable for public consumption. Water drawn from sources that are substantially pollution free, such as deep ground-waters in rural areas or upland water from areas with no public access, normally require no or minimal treatment apart from final disinfection with chlorine. At the opposite extreme, water from the lowland

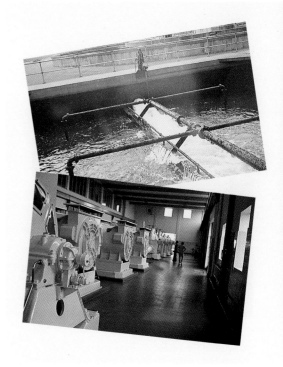

Water treatment plant.

Figure 2.11
In a conventional water treatment plant, water is filtered, treated with chemicals to remove fine particles and then disinfected with chlorine.

KEY:
1: Chemical mixing basin   ⎫ Coagulation and
2: Flocculation basin   ⎬ Flocculation
3: Settling tank
4: Rapid sand filter
5: Disinfection with chlorine
6: Clean water storage basin (Clear well)
7: Pump

reaches of a river, containing a high proportion of sewage and industrial effluent, needs extensive treatment to be rendered wholesome and aesthetically pleasing. Figure 2.11 summarizes the treatment processes used in purification of the public water supply, and shows the layout of a typical, conventional water treatment works.

Water treatment plants clarify the water so that disinfection can be effectively carried out. The two major methods in use are:

1 Conventional treatment.

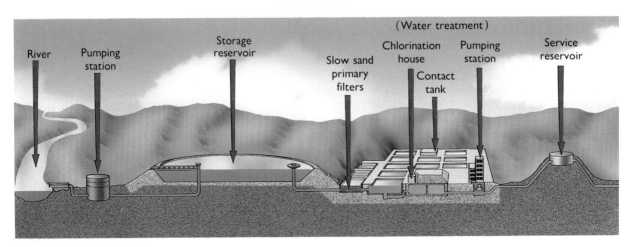

2 Slow sand filtration.

Figure 2.12
Slow sand filtration removes bacteria and suspended materials by the biological action of micro-organisms living on the surface of the sand.

Conventional treatment involves screening the water, adjusting the pH (acidity or alkalinity), adding coagulation chemicals such as aluminium sulphate or iron salts, flocculation to remove very fine particles, then rapid filtration through sand or multi-media (anthracite, sand, activated carbon) and finally disinfection with chlorine. Where special problems may occur, ozone or

Parameter	Unit	EEC Directive 1980	WHO Guidelines 1984	Water Supply (Water Quality) Regulations 1989
Total coliforms	MPN/100ml	Nil	3	Nil
Faecal coliforms	MPN/100ml	Nil	Nil	Nil
Total solids	mg/l	1500	1000	1500
Iron	µg/l	200	300	200
Copper	µg/l	3000	1000	3000
Zinc	µg/l	5000	5000	5000
Arsenic	µg/l	50	50	50
Lead	µg/l	50	50	50
Mercury	µg/l	1	1	1
Phenol	µg/l	0.5	N/A	0.5
Surfactants	µg/l MBAS	200	–	200
Chlorides	mg/l	400	250	400
Nitrates	mg/l NO_3	50	44	50
Nitrites	mg/l NO_2	0.1	N/A	0.1
THM	µg/l	N/A	–	100
Chloroform	µg/l	N/A	30	100
Pesticides	µg/l	0.5	0.03–30	0.5
DDT	µg/l	0.1	1	0.1
PAH	µg/l	0.2	0.2	0.2

Table 2.1
Comparison of water quality standards

Source: A Report on a London-wide Survey of Drinking Water Quality. Berridge Environmental Laboratories Ltd. 1990

chlorine dioxide are used early in the process to disinfect the supplies. Increasingly, activated carbon is being used as a polishing treatment to remove organics such as pesticides and taste- and odour-producing chemicals. Similarly, the use of aluminium is being more closely monitored, even being replaced by iron salt coagulants. Control of water supplies is continually being improved to produce tap water that is free of bacteria and organics and which is not corrosive or scale-forming.

Slow sand filtration relies on the slow passage of water through a fine grade of sand (Figure 2.12). Biological processes at the surface of the sand remove bacteria and suspended material. No chemicals need be added except at the end of the treatment to disinfect the supply.

Additional treatment options such as softening, hardening, iron and manganese removal and fluoridation can be used according to the needs of the consumer. All water supplies are required to meet the specifications of the Water Supply (Water Quality) Regulations 1989 (Table 2.1). The impact of privatisation on water supplies has been to increase their concern for the quality of services provided to the consumer.

Closer control is being exercised on industrial pollution and leachate from solid and toxic waste sites contaminating water, as a result of stronger public awareness created by environmental pressure groups. This is as much a matter of saving on costs of cleansing water supplies as of environmental concern. Closer monitoring by the National Rivers Authority and the River Purification Boards in Scotland will hopefully improve conditions in UK rivers. As the nature of industry changes, the type

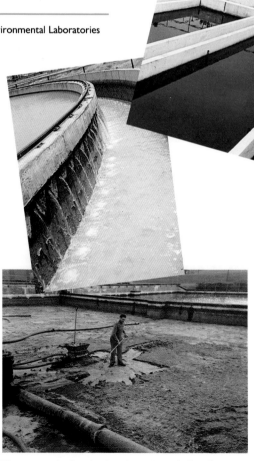

The amount of water treatment needed varies greatly depending on its source.

and quality of effluent discharges will alter. The 'policing' of industrial waste discharge will still need to be intense, and provision of sufficient inspectorate staff and facilities will have to be maintained for proper surveillance.

A major problem for water supply companies is to reduce losses in distribution systems. Up to 40% of treated, pumped water may leak out of the system owing to the poor condition of pipes, tanks and reservoirs. If pressures are reduced too much, dirty water can be sucked back into the pipes. Pipes are often up to 100 years old and may be made of poor quality iron which has been corroded by aggressive water inside and aggressive soils outside. Old distribution pipes are being renovated with cement mortar or epoxy internal relining, or are being replaced with plastic pipes. These improvements increase the cost of water to the consumer, particularly as they have to be carried out with minimum disruption to supplies and to road traffic.

The UK water industry will be spending £1.4 billion at 1987/88 prices over the next 5 years on their programmes. For some pesticides the limit in the EC Directive is not currently achievable by any member state because the technology for full-scale treatment is not yet sufficiently developed or because effective solutions have not yet been found.

The effect of privatization has been to increase concern for the customer, so the search for new, more effective and less costly chemical removal methods continues. An interesting new development has been the use in the USA of crown ethers to clean up water supplies polluted by toxic metals such as lead, mercury, cadmium and zinc. The process involves molecules called crown ethers, whose structure enables them to 'seize' metal ions. The new process is of particular interest to battery companies and film processors, whose industries discharge a lot of lead and other metals – such as arsenic, nickel, chromium, antimony and copper – in their effluent. Also in the USA, engineers in California claim to have developed a form of steam cleaning that removes petrochemicals from contaminated soil. By injecting steam into highly contaminated soil in California's Silicon Valley, the engineers say that they are able to remove 99.5% of the pollutants from soil and ground-water. The steam heats the soil causing the pollutants to vaporize. The team has managed to remove 14 different organic compounds, including trichloroethylene, acetone, and xylene.

CHEMICALS IN SOIL

This chapter has concentrated on the impact of chemicals on water and the aquatic biota. Before we leave chemicals in the environment it is necessary to look briefly at the ways in which chemicals can enter the soil and thence pass into the water supply (Figure 2.13). There is also a risk to human health from chemicals ingested in food grown on contaminated soil, through ingestion of the soil itself and through indirect absorption following contact between soil and the skin. It is more likely that some pesticides will be eaten with the plant than absorbed from the drinking water.

There are four main pathways by which a chemical in the soil can enter a plant[63]. These are:

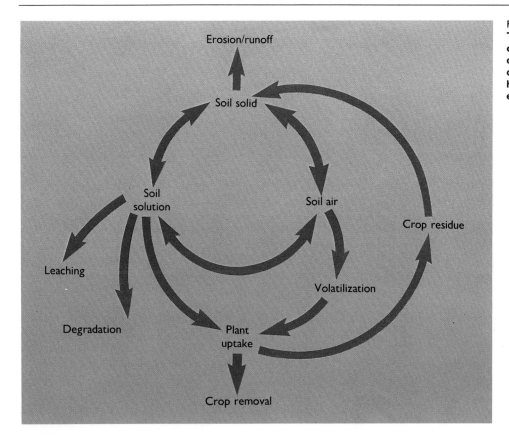

Erosion/runoff

Soil solid

Soil air

Crop residue

Soil solution

Leaching

Volatilization

Degradation

Plant uptake

Crop removal

Figure 2.13
The characteristics of a chemical determine its distribution in soil, its degradation rate and hence its impact on the environment.

1 Root uptake and subsequent upward movement in the plant.
2 Uptake of vapour from the surrounding air.
3 Uptake by external contamination of shoots by soil and dust, followed by retention in the plant cuticle or penetration through it.
4 Uptake and transportation in oil-containing cells found in plants like carrots and cress.

Chemicals can contaminate the soil in a variety of ways, some deliberate, some accidental. Examples of soil contamination include:

1 Spills which can result from overfilling of containers or design faults.
2 Accidents including rail and road traffic accidents, or industrial process failures which lead to an escape of material (for example, the Seveso incident in Northern Italy in 1976, Bhopal in India, Coalite plant in Derbyshire).
3 Leakage, which may occur undetected for long periods from underground pipelines on tanks (for example, Mildenhall in 1981).
4 Storage of coal for example, which on bare earth can produce significant contamination.
5 Waste disposal (see *landfill* above).
6 Use of products such as fertilizers which are deliberately added to the soil[25].

The dichotomy between the benefits of pesticides and the possible risks to human health from their presence in soil serves to remind us of the difficult balance between risk and benefit which is central to any discussion of chemicals in the environment.

ENVIRONMENTAL CONTROLS

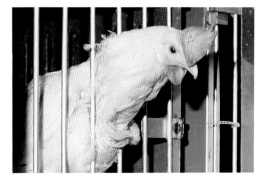

Intensive rearing of poultry produces highly polluting liquors.

Potent chemicals and toxic substances are readily available to the amateur gardener.

Chemicals reach the water environment in many ways: by solution of substances from the atmosphere, by run-off and infiltration from the land, industrial and toxic waste discharges and, not least, domestic sewage and wastewater. In a highly industrialized and populated country such as the UK, spillage accidents will occur despite good intentions and controls. New chemicals are constantly being produced that add to the variety of chemicals being found in the environment. Changes in agricultural practice, such as intensive rearing of cattle, poultry, sheep and pigs, silage-making which produces highly polluting liquors, and increased use of fertilizers can create potential water contamination problems. Pesticides and herbicides are not only used by farmers, but also by local authorities on roadside verges, by British Rail on embankments and cuttings, by electricity boards under pylons and by the domestic gardener in his allotment and garden.

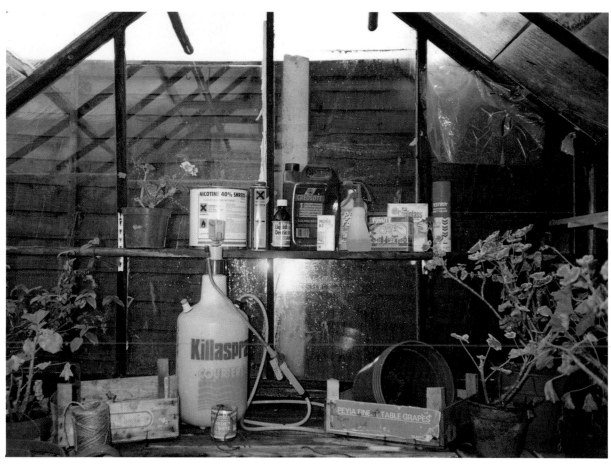

Advances in analytical techniques have allowed measurement of very low levels of chemicals. Some of the chemicals detected at these levels have toxic properties at much higher concentrations, so their mere presence in water has created concern. The National Rivers Authority in England and Wales and the River Purification Boards in Scotland have statutory powers to protect water supplies from pollutants by imposing tight controls on man-made discharges. Industrialists and the farming community can also adopt more responsible environmental attitudes, especially in respect of ground-water pollution.

Treatment technology is changing rapidly to reduce levels of lead, pesticides, aluminium and aggressive water. In a letter to the European Commission dated 16 November 1989, the Department of the Environment issued a programme for improving drinking water standards. The main points were as follows:

'Improvement programmes of water service companies in England and Wales would bring virtually all drinking water supplies up to standard by 1995. This includes the standards for aluminium, nitrate and lead.'

The customer buying water from a water company has the power to demand better quality in what is a 'food grade' product. Investment is needed to rehabilitate old distribution systems to prevent leakage and stop dirty water entering the mains. This will provide a more attractive product without resort to home filter systems or very expensive bottled waters.

Public confidence depends upon improvements in water quality. Environmental pressure groups are having an effect on attitudes in the UK. EC legislation has generated pressure for improvements in water quality and supply. The key to the improvement of water quality is pollution prevention.

The increasing popularity of bottled waters reflects public concern over the quality of tap water.

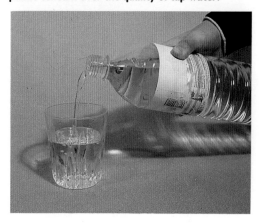

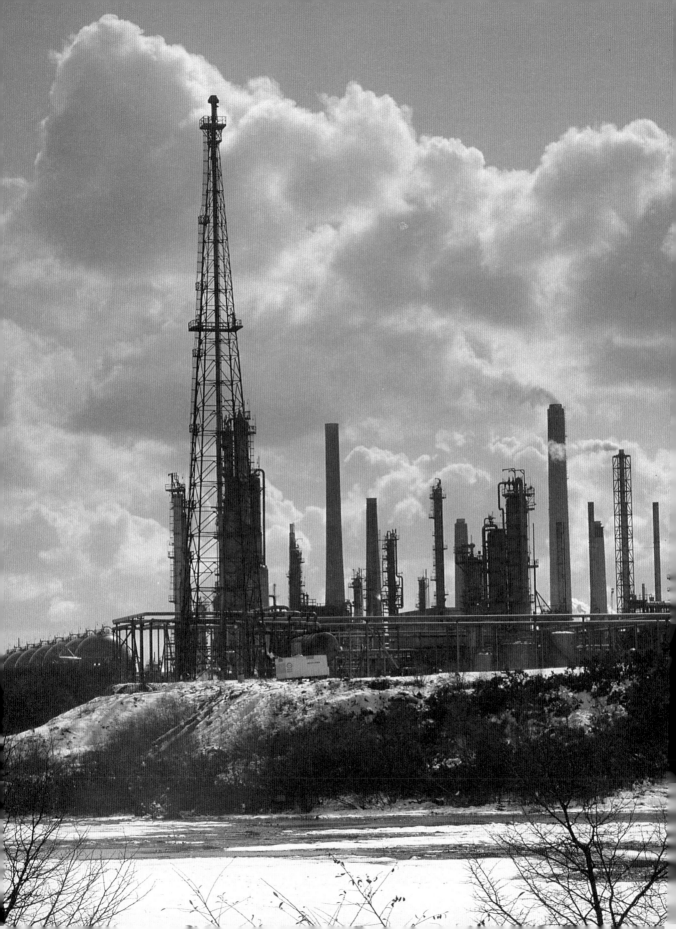

3 PESTICIDE MANUFACTURE AND TESTING

So what are pesticides, how are they made and tested, how are they stored and transported, and who buys them? Having examined the historical, political and ecological context of chemicals in the environment, we now turn more specifically to pesticides and their uses.

CONSTITUENTS AND FORMULATION

Any pesticide is a mixture of ingredients including not only the active ingredient but also the additives that go to make it a usable formulated product.

The *active ingredient* is the basic chemical that kills or controls the pest or pests. It is known by its chemical name (for example tetramethylthiuram disulphide) and almost invariably has a Chemical Abstracts Registration Number or CAS RN (a number like 137-26-8). The active ingredient usually has a common name, in this case thiram.

The *formulated product* is the active ingredient plus other chemicals used to formulate it, made up into the commercial, ready-to-use product, sold under a brand name, or variety of names. These additional chemicals might include:

1 *Solvents* – Chemicals used to formulate the product (for example, make it into a liquid). Many pesticides are now water based.
2 *Surfactants* – Comprising wetters, spreaders and some stickers (surfactants is short for surface active agents). They help to reduce the surface tension, increasing the emulsifying, spreading and wetting properties of liquid formulations. Surfactants are not necessarily stated on the label.
3 *Carriers* – Liquid or solid substances added to a pesticide to dilute it to facilitate its application. Carriers are not necessarily stated on the label.
4 *Safeners* – Chemicals that reduce the potential of a pesticide to harm the crop itself. Safeners are not necessarily stated on the label.
5 *Adjuvants* – Chemicals added to a pesticide to increase its efficiency. Adjuvants are inactive without the presence of the pesticide active ingredient.

Pesticides can be sold in a number of different forms, broadly divided into liquid and powder formulations:

1 Liquid formulations can be:
   (a) *Emulsifiable concentrate (EC)* – a homogeneous liquid formulation which forms an emulsion on mixing with water.

(b) *Emulsion* – A mixture in which fine globules of one liquid are dispersed in another.

(c) *Suspension concentrate (SC)* – A stable suspension of finely ground active ingredient(s) in water intended for dilution before use.

2 Solid formulations can be:

(a) *Water-soluble powder* – a powder formulation which forms a true solution of the active ingredients when dissolved in water.

(b) *Wettable powder (water dispersible powder)* – A powder formulation which is dispersible in water to form a suspension.

(c) *Grains* – Granular or grain-like pellets which contain or are coated with the active ingredient.

A single active ingredient can occur in many brand-named products. For example, thiram (a fungicide) is marketed under its own name by several companies, but also appears under the following product names: Cunitex, General Garden Fungicide, Hy-Vic, Tripomol 80 and Soluble. It is also mixed with other chemicals and sold as H115, Hydra-Guard, New Hydra-Guard, New Hysede, Hytal, Gammalax Liquid, Vitavax, Brassica Collar, Flora Spray, Secto Garden Powder, Systemic Insecticide Fungicide Rose and Flower Spray, Turbair Botry-cide, Mist-O-Matic Lindex Plus FS Seed Treatment, Boots Spring and Autumn Lawn Treatment, and Green Fingers Hormone Rooting Powder.

PESTICIDE PRODUCTION

Pesticide manufacture is dominated by large chemical companies – American, British, German, Swiss, Italian, Dutch and Japanese (Table 3.1). Some of these companies (such as ICI or Dow-Elanco) have interests in a wide range of chemical products. Many also produce pharmaceutical products (for

Company	1976	1983	1985	1987	
				Rank	Sales ($b)
Ciba Geigy	2	2	2	1	2.0
Bayer*	1	1	1	2	2.0
ICI*	10	5	4	3	1.8
Rhone Poulenc*	4	6	6	4	1.6
Du Pont*	9	8	10	5	1.2
Monsato	4	3	3	6	1.2
Shell*	3	4	5	7	1.0
BASF	7	9	7	8	1.0
Hoechst	12	7	8	9	0.9
Dow	16	10	9	10	0.8

$b = Billions (1000 million) of dollars
*Involved in major acquisitions and/or divestments during the period.
Source: County NatWest WoodMac, in World Crop Protection Prospects: Demisting the Crystal Ball. The Bawden Memorial Lecture, Brighton Crop Protection Conference, 1988

Table 3.1
Agrochemical companies: world ranking

example, Rhone-Poulenc, Hoechst, and ICI). There are also a number of smaller manufacturers who produce off-patent 'commodity' pesticides. The research and development costs of producing chemicals such as pesticides are now so high that only large companies can afford to undertake the ever-increasing safety tests. The development of fewer, but much larger, companies may have been motivated by profit, but this has also led to higher safety standards.

For some years the leading position in the world ranking of agrochemical companies was held by Bayer. However, following a period of major acquisition and disinvestment by many of the leading companies, Ciba Geigy assumed the title in 1987, with worldwide sales totalling $2 billion. The number of European based companies in the top ten in the USA has increased from two in 1980 to five in 1987. Increasingly, Japanese companies are finding their way onto the international stage[64].

The pesticides industry is part of a larger organic chemical industry. In the words of the US National Institute for Occupational Safety and Health (NIOSH), the industry structure is pyramid shaped, with hundreds of manufacturers, thousands of formulators, and millions of users[65]. Pesticide production is a two stage process: manufacturing and formulation. The manufacturing process produces the active pesticide ingredient by chemical synthetic procedures. The active ingredients are then transformed into formulated products by dissolving them in solvents, mixing them with carriers and so on, as already described.

One disturbing aspect of pesticide production is the possible use of agrochemical plants to manufacture chemical agents that could be used in human warfare. At an physiological level, there is no real difference between insects, or other pests, and humans in terms of their nervous systems. Factories used in the making of pesticides may need only slight modifications to enable them to manufacture substances used in human warfare. Because of this concern, chemicals that could be used in this way, such as phosphorus oxichloride, require special licences for export. In discussing the risks of pesticides to human health, the possibility that the legitimate production of pesticides may be subject to abuse should not be overlooked. It is therefore essential that effective international agreements should be enforced to control the production of these hazardous chemicals.

MANUFACTURING PROCESSES

Pesticide manufacture is carried out in relatively few plants. In general, a few pesticides are produced at each plant and a few plants produce each pesticide. Employees include chemists, engineers, chemical operators, pipefitters, electricians and labourers.

Originally, the production of agrochemicals was a simple process, often by the reaction of two readily available organic molecules to produce another, which had a pesticidal activity. However, as agrochemicals have become more specific and selective, the complexity of the molecules has increased with a consequent increase in the number of stages of production.

When people think of the chemical industry they envisage large installations, such as refineries. Refineries are extremely complicated pieces of engineering which operate more or less continuously to produce a small range of chemical products from a small range of inputs. The production of agrochemicals rarely takes place in such complex, continuous process plants. Agrochemicals are produced mainly in batches, with perhaps only one or two stages occurring in the reaction process of each batch, involving perhaps only a tonne of material. Many active ingredients are produced in small quantities, and of the 1000 or so active ingredients worldwide only a handful are made in quantities greater than 1000 tonnes annually. The processes used in the manufacture of active ingredients in pesticides vary a good deal, but broadly there are the following stages[66,67]:

1 *Raw materials* are delivered in bulk by rail, road, pipeline and so on, or may be produced within the plant. Examples of these materials are ammonia, benzene, bromine, chlorine, formaldehyde, phenol and sulphuric acid.
2 *Production of the pesticidal chemical* is the next stage. In the processing of 'natural' pesticides such as pyrethrum, refining is the only step. Otherwise production begins with *synthesis* of the pesticide in a single or multi-step chemical process.
3 *Separation* of the pesticide from by-products, solvents, and unreacted ingredients then takes place. This is performed by various equipment including filters and centrifuges. The separated materials will inevitably contain some residual pesticide, so great care needs to be taken in their disposal or re-use.

Another purification stage usually follows, using centrifuges, stills, evaporators and driers. In some cases the impurities removed at this stage may pose a greater hazard to workers than the pesticide itself.

Pesticide manufacturing operations in the UK are subject to the Health and Safety at Work etc Act 1974, to the Control of Substances Hazardous to Health (COSHH) Regulations 1989 and to periodic visits by inspectors from the Health and Safety Executive (HSE). Most of the major producers employ their own toxicologists, occupational hygienists, safety engineers, occupational physicians and nurses to ensure that employees are subjected to minimum risks from chemical exposures. Controlled emissions from manufacturing processes are subject to the Control of Pollution Act (1974) and Water Act (1989), and may be restricted further in future 'Green' legislation.

FORMULATION PROCESSES

Pesticides are rarely, if ever, applied to the crop in the form in which they are delivered from the plant carrying out the synthesis. The products at this stage are often viscous or solid materials which would be impossible to apply by farm machinery. A process called formulation therefore needs to be undertaken, with the objective of producing a product that can be applied by the farmer. The principal methods of application are in the form of solid granule or liquid spray.

The formulating process is generally less complex than the manufacturing operation. Usually a formulator receives concentrated active ingredients from a manufacturer or customer and dilutes them with various non-pesticide materials known as 'inerts'. While inerts are taken into account in the evaluation of the hazards of a pesticide formulation, some are more toxic to man than the name would suggest. The potential hazards of these so-called inert ingredients of pesticide products have been pointed out by the Residues Sub-Group of the Government's Research Consultative Committee which reported in 1988. This group stated that: 'Although these inert substances may be minor components of the formulation many exhibit significant mammalian toxicities ... the attention of the sub-group was drawn to increasing concern about those substances'[40]. These substances have been classified into four toxicity categories (see Federal Register Vol 52, No 77, 13305). The formulation process may also include physical or chemical treatment to produce particular product forms (powders, aerosols, pellets). Several active ingredients may be included in the final product, widening its usefulness to the farmer. In addition, stabilizers (agents to cause the ingredient to be more adherent to the crop) and warning agents such as dyes or stenches may be incorporated.

As with pesticide manufacture, formulation plants are subject to the control of the Health and Safety at Work etc Act (1974) and COSHH (1989).

The final stage of the process involves the packaging and labelling of the product, prior to its entering the distribution chain. Depending on customer requirements, pesticides may be packaged in a variety of containers ranging from small glass or plastic bottles to railway wagons. The type of packaging is obviously also dependent on the final product form – that is, powder, liquid, gas and so on. The packaging may be carried out at the plant, sometimes with automatic dispensing, weighing and sealing equipment. Packaging is also carried out by the formulators and sometimes by specialist packers. The package size of agrochemicals is often small, with quantities of 50 or 100 ml for domestic use, and 1–10 litres for agricultural use. Powders are often supplied in 1–5 kg packs. In the case of both liquids and powders, packs of 25 or 200 litres are occasionally produced. Good package design is an important factor in reducing the incidence of spillage and splashing by operators.

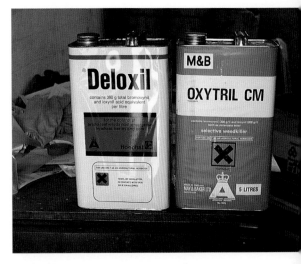

Pesticides should be packaged in well-designed containers, which are clearly labelled.

PREVENTION AND CONTROL MEASURES

A wide variety of substances hazardous to health, ranging from the pesticide active ingredient(s) to chemical solvents, are used in the manufacture and formulation of the ready-to-use product.

Those involved in manufacture and formulation face a correspondingly wide range of acute and chronic health hazards. These range from irritant skin and respiratory effects to more serious, long-term problems such as the well-documented link between exposure to the pesticide DCBP and reproductive hazards[68]. It is important, therefore, that there is proper risk assessment of hazards, carried out by 'competent', trained and/

or qualified personnel, and that the appropriate prevention and control and checking measures, such as health surveillance, are implemented.

Because of the contained nature of the processes it is often easier to control hazards in the manufacturing/formulation sector than with use. Control measures include enclosed/contained processes, local exhaust ventilation, and safe disposal procedures linked to proper training of the workforce. Control measures should be regularly checked to see that they are working by means of planned maintenance and environmental monitoring to measure airborne concentrations of chemicals, as well as by health surveillance of the workforce.

One problem noted by the HSE is the variability of the setting of Occupational Exposure Limits (OELs) between different pesticide manufacturers and even between different plants owned by the same company. OEL's are maximum (not safe) airborne concentrations of chemicals, which the employer must not exceed and, indeed, must try to reduce exposure to below these levels. If too high an OEL is set then the workforce could be exposed to preventable health hazards.

The number of legally determined OELs is limited and manufacturers must determine and set their own limits for many chemicals. The HSE is worried about how this is done and what criteria manufacturers use in determining health risk in setting the limits. It is trying to help standardize the setting of OELs in pesticide manufacturing and formulation. The COSHH Regulations 1988 should lead to improvements in the setting of OELs and other prevention and control measures in chemical plants.

Manufacturers have responsibilities not only to safeguard the health of their own workforce, but also to protect users of their products, wildlife and the environment. This can be achieved by ensuring that products, including tank mixes, are properly researched and tested; and that full health and safety information is provided to users, including summaries of the main data in an easily understood form. This is especially important for chronic health risks, and for older pesticides which have not been tested to modern safety standards. Such research, testing and provision of information is a legal requirement under Section 6 of the Health and Safety at Work etc Act 1974 as amended by the Consumer Protection Act 1987.

Pesticide manufacturers also have clear responsibilities with regard to the export of pesticides, given the large number of deaths and poisonings from pesticide use in developing countries. Export controls to developing countries should be strengthened and manufacturers should play a more active role in ensuring that their products are used more safely in such areas of the world.

TESTING AND PRODUCT DEVELOPMENT

In the competitive climate of agrochemicals the search for new products is intense. The stakes are high and there is huge investment in research and development before a product goes onto the market. In 1987 it was estimated that the cost of developing a new pesticide was approximately $45 million dollars. A new pesticide probably requires the screening of 20000 or more chemicals before a successful product can be identified. The development of a new pesticide chemical, from discovery to full marketing, usually spans from 8–10 years. During this period three areas of activity go on in parallel. There are the manufacturing aspects (including the scaling up of production from laboratory synthesis to manufacturing scale, the development of preferred formulations, and patent claims); the biological aspects (including defining the areas of recommended use and limitations); and the product safety aspects. Product safety includes the health of the manufacturing worker and the final user, the overall environmental safety, and the safety of those who consume the treated crops (including livestock animals as well as human). The safety aspects of manufacture, formulation, packing, transport and use of the pesticide, as well as disposal of the used container, are all examined.

In order to discover a new pesticide it is estimated that approximately 25000 new compounds must be synthesized to produce just one product. New pesticides must meet the criteria of safety, economy and efficacy. The industry estimate for the costs of development of a single product is approximately £12 million. To this should be added the research and development costs for all the new compounds that were shown ultimately to be unsuccessful. If such costs are included, the true total for the development of a single new product is around £60 million.

A significant portion of the costs towards development is related to safety testing. In order to obtain the approval of government regulatory bodies a number of 'core' studies must be undertaken which in themselves cost about £2.5 million for a single crop use. In addition, individual governments have further specific safety requirements which must be satisfied, and these pose additional costs of up to £1 million.

Typically the safety programmes take a minimum of 6 years to complete before the data are comprehensive enough for submission to governments to obtain registration. Many candidate products are eliminated during this development period because they do not meet the necessary criteria. Tables 3.2–3.4 show the scope of the core studies currently required for registration purposes in the areas of mammalian toxicology, environmental studies and residue studies.

An extensive series of pre-marketing tests are carried out, using animal experiments (chiefly with rats, mice, rabbits and guinea pigs). Although there is always controversy about animal experiments, there seems at the moment to be little real alternative if a high degree of pesticide safety is to be assured. It is in the industry's own interests to avoid duplication of toxicity tests, and this at the very least ensures that the minimum number of tests are carried out on the minimum numbers of animals.

In 1982 Roberts[69] produced the following summary of the stages in pesticide development and toxicological testing. Since then there have been some changes but the general outline is still valid. All major companies now evaluate, prior to development, many of the analogues of a chemical series so that only those promising compounds, with the least potential for effects on health and the environment, go forward for development:

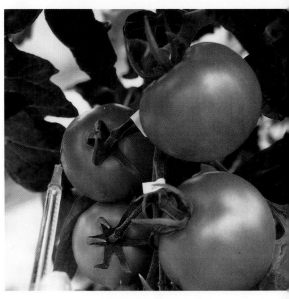

Before they are allowed to be marketed, pesticides must undergo rigorous testing.

Year 1 – Acute tests on a new technical pesticide begin. There may be further evaluations, particularly if the synthetic pathway changes and new formulations appear.

Year 2 – Acute tests on trial formulations begin; these may be extended into the third year.

Year 3 – Short-term (90-day) animal studies begin and end. Animal metabolism tests begin and go on into a fourth year. Teratogenicity and mutagenicity tests begin at this phase if they have not been tested at an earlier screening level.

Year 4 – Start of major 2-year mouse, 2-year rat and 1-year dog studies, which go on into the sixth year. Reproduction, teratogenic and genotoxicity studies continue.

Year 5 – Major biotransformation studies.

Year 6 – No new studies, but continuation of animal studies and studies in metabolism. The application for permission to use the compound is made.

Year 7 – Registration of the product is obtained, and marketing commences. Supporting investigatory studies in response to regulatory queries and additional studies to explain or assess any human health impact of a toxicological finding in animals are all taking place, and will continue during the life of a product.

As in the pharmaceutical industry, the financial commitment of the company is clearly considerable before detailed health and safety tests relating to long-term risks begin. Only about 25% of compounds entering the final phase will actually achieve full commercialisation. The others are withdrawn on safety grounds, following the results of toxicity and environmental testing.

PESTICIDE APPROVAL

Any pesticide active ingredient or formulated product must now be vetted and approved by the Government's Approvals Scheme. Under the Food and Environment Protection Act (1985) it is now illegal to sell, supply, store, advertise, or use a pesticide unless it has received approval. The Act is implemented through the Control of Pesticides Regulations 1986 (COPR), which have replaced the non-statutory Pesticides Safety Precautions Scheme (PSPS). MAFF has issued draft Codes of Practice on Agricultural and Commercial Horticultural Use of Pesticides and on Storage, Sale and Supply of Pesticides. The codes provide guidance on how to fulfil the requirements of the 1985 Act, although failure to follow this guidance does not in itself constitute an offence; a failure to do so can be used as evidence in criminal proceedings.

Under the new regulations pesticides may be granted:

1 An experimental permit, which enables testing and development work to be carried out.
2 A provisional approval for a limited period.
3 A full approval for an unstipulated period.

A company intending to market a new pesticide or recommend a new use for an existing product must submit data to the registration authority (the Pesticides Safety Division of MAFF, or in some cases the HSE). Applicants must provide enough data to enable an assessment to be made of whether the product may be used safely, and includes:

1 Information on the physical and chemical properties of the *active ingredient* (Table 3.2).

Acute and dose–range finding studies AI	Subchronic studies AI	Chronic studies AI	Studies on proposed AI formulations
Oral and dermal acutes, irritancy and skin sensitization tests	3-month repeat dose studies in rodents and non-rodents	2-year rat and mouse studies for long-term effects	Oral and dermal acutes, irritancy and skin sensitization tests. Ames test
Preliminary mutagenicity testing – Ames test	Teratology in two species	I year non-rodent	Dermal penetration study (or studies) in rats
Repeat dose range finding studies in two species, up to I month	Inhalation if appropriate	Rat reproduction (two or three generation)	
	ADME studies		
	Further mutagenicity testing		

Table 3.2
Numbers of documented cases of insecticide resistance

AI = Active ingredient; ADME = absorbtion, distribution, metabolism and excretion.

2 Information on the *formulated product* and its application.
3 *Residue studies* (Table 3.3).
4 Data on *toxicity in animals*, including acute toxicity, sub-acute and short-term toxicity, metabolism of the product, delayed effects, long-term toxicity, carcinogenicity, teratogenicity and mutagenicity studies.
5 *Environmental studies* (Table 3.4) to determine any short- or long-term effects of the pesticide on wildlife, which includes laboratory and field studies on fish and the aquatic environment, birds, mammals, bees, flora, and beneficial insects and soil organisms.

Table 3.3
Residue and metabolism studies: plant metabolism

Crop residue active ingredient and metabolite
Lactating ruminant study
Ruminant tissue study
Poultry metabolism and residue
Residues in crops harvested and processed
Taint (as appropriate)

Wildlife toxicity	Environmental fate
Earthworm	Plant metabolism
Honey-bee	Soil respiration
Daphnia	Soil nitrification
Daphnia long-term	Soil ammonification
Algae	Soil aerobic metabolism
Carp	Soil anaerobic metabolism
Rainbow trout	Sterile soil metabolism
Fish	Soil adsorption/desorption
Fish long-term study	Soil leaching
Beneficial insects	Aged soil leaching
	Crop rotation
	Aqueous and soil photolysis
	Hydrolysis study

Table 3.4
Environmental studies for pesticide approval

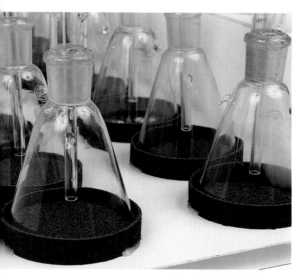

Samples of soil are studied to measure residue levels of a new pesticide and its effect on beneficial insects and soil organisms.

After evaluating the data, and providing they are acceptable, the independent Advisory Committee on Pesticides makes recommendations on whether the component should be approved for use, the level of approval, and the safety precautions and conditions of use.

Acting on these recommendations, Ministers may grant an approval. All approvals are subject to review at any time in the light of new evidence. In addition, all pesticides are subject to full scientific reviews 10 years from the date of the first commercial approval of the active ingredient. The authorities have the right to require further toxicological or environmental tests or can require that the entire toxicological package be carried out again. Reviews will be repeated at 10-year intervals for as long as the product is on the market[70].

Although the new regulatory system is now in operation, the agrochemical industry and pressure groups have both expressed concern at the delays in obtaining registrations for new products and in implementing safety reviews. The British Agrochemicals Association (BAA) points to the loss of exports that can result from delays in registration of UK products, as well as the disadvantage at which this places UK farmers. The backlogs can also slow down the registration and availability of new, less toxic and more environmentally friendly pesticides. MAFF has a list of over 100 long established pesticides awaiting safety reviews because they were not subjected to modern safety analysis before approval. These include the commonly used fungicides maneb, mancozeb and zineb, which are currently being investigated by the US Environmental Protection Agency. Following pressure from the industry and environmentalists, the Minister of Agriculture announced in April 1990 an increase of staff at the MAFF Pesticides Registration Section and a contracting out of routine work in an attempt to clear backlogs.

These issues were addressed in a series of meetings organized by the Green Alliance during 1989, which included representatives of the BAA, Friends of the Earth, the Transport and General Workers Union, the Pesticides Trust and the National Federation of Women's Institutes. On 7 August 1989 the group issued a joint letter to Government ministers responsible for pesticides, proposing five reforms:

1 The organizations welcomed the programme of regular reviews of older pesticides, but felt that a 10-year timescale was not acceptable. It was believed that 1992 would be a more appropriate target for completing these reviews, and that this would require a tripling of resources.
2 So that newer, safer pesticides were able to clear the system and replace older less benign chemicals, a reduction in the waiting time for approval of new pesticides to 1 year was suggested.
3 Provision should be made for the appointment of at least 100 extra Health and Safety Inspectors to ensure that pesticide regulations were properly enforced. The Institution of Professional Civil Servants estimates that the average farm is visited only once in 9.8 years, and a self-employed farmer might not see an inspector for 29 years. This cannot be conducive to effective enforcement of the regulations.

4 There should be more frequent testing for pesticide residues over a broader range of foodstuffs.

5 A single national pesticide incidents monitoring scheme should be set up to replace the four different systems operated by the HSE, the Department of Trade and Industry, the Department of Health, and the National Poisons Information Centres.

The results from the single monitoring scheme should be made easily accessible to the public. The development of these areas of agreement between the agrochemical industry (which has offered to pay for increased resources for pesticide registration), environmentalists, trade unionists and representatives of consumers and the community, is encouraging evidence of an emerging consensus on practical improvements in the testing and use of pesticides.

ACCIDENTS DURING MANUFACTURE AND FORMULATION

Manufacturing of any chemical can be a dangerous procedure, whether it is a medicine, explosive, pesticide or one of many other compounds which are being produced. The safety record of the chemical industry in the UK is among the highest in industry and pesticide manufacturers take their responsibilities very seriously, doing all they can to minimize risk. However, there have been cases where the risks have been underestimated or ignored. Such lapses can go unnoticed – until there is a major disaster.

Such a disaster occurred on the night of 2 December 1984, in Bhopal, India. Bhopal is an industrial town of 800 000 people in Northern India. In 1969 the chemical company Union Carbide began building a chemical plant. Initially this was a plant for mixing, dilution and packaging of imported chemicals (a formulation plant), but in 1980 it developed into a full scale manufacturing unit. The main product was carbaryl, a carbamate pesticide usually sold under the name of Sevin. One of the raw materials used in the production of carbaryl is methyl isocyanate (MIC), a substance that is acutely toxic by inhalation.

The Bhopal disaster occurred when water entered a storage tank, causing polymerization of the MIC. The subsequent rise in pressure caused 30 tonnes of MIC to escape from the tank. It is estimated that a quarter of the population of Bhopal, some 200 000 people, inhaled the gas. The official death tally 2 years later registered 2352 deaths, although this is almost certainly an underestimate. Thousands more are still suffering adverse health effects, including lung damage and eye disorders. Although the precise details of death toll and injury will never be known, Bhopal was undoubtedly a disaster of unprecedented proportions. Such large scale disasters are not representative of the prevailing standards in manufacturing practice in the developed world. The high number of deaths at Bhopal was a consequence of the growth of a shanty town around the factory. However, there is no place for complacency about safety standards, even in the western world.

A serious chemical manufacturing accident occurred at Seveso in Italy in 1976. A chemical plant owned by Givaudan, a subsidiary of the Swiss pharmaceutical company Hoffman-La Roche, was involved in the manufacture of an intermediate used to make the bactericide hexachlorophene (a pharmaceutical, not pesticidal, product). The chemical intermediate in question was 2,4,5-trichlorophenol, which was being produced at the time of the accident. A vat at the plant exploded, releasing a chemical cloud over 18 km^2 of the surrounding countryside. The cloud consisted primarily of sodium trichlorophenate, but also contained a quantity of the by-product 2,3,7,8-tetrachlorodibenzo-p-dioxin (dioxin)[71]. Seven hundred people were evacuated some 2 weeks after the accident, and many people in the vacated area and the residential neighbourhood area to the south of the factory had been exposed to toxic chemicals. Immediate effects were burns and facial swelling in children caused by the caustic sodium trichlorophenate, but any long-term health effects have been difficult to assess because of difficulties in collecting data.

Following the accident the Lombardy Region mounted an extensive health surveillance programme. All those at risk were monitored, although there was no provision for a comparable control group. About 200 children developed chloracne (it was argued that children were outside more and therefore more exposed to dioxin), but by 1978 their condition had improved markedly. Subsequent tests showed no apparent immunological damage in these children.

There was an increase in congenital malformations recorded in 1977 and 1978 which may have been due to the effects of dioxin poisoning, but could equally well have been the result of more diligent reporting. Having been made aware of the risks posed by dioxin, physicians became more reliable in reporting any abnormalities they observed[72-75]. Dioxin is extremely toxic to certain animals, and exposure to dioxin in the Seveso incident indicated a prevalence of chloracne in children up to 14 years of age. The toxicity of dioxin to human beings is not clear, and the UK Government's Committee on Toxicity of Chemicals in Food, Consumer Products and the Environment has not been able to set a definitive acceptable daily intake of dioxins for humans[76].

Seveso gave its name to the EC 'Seveso Directive' aimed at large-scale disaster planning in industrial processes. The Directive has been implemented in the UK by the Control of Industrial Major Hazards Regulations 1984 known as CIMAH. CIMAH requires those in control of activities involving dangerous substances to demonstrate to HSE that major accident hazards have been recognized, that measures have been taken to prevent accidents and to minimize the consequences should they occur, and to report any major accidents.

A serious ecological disaster occurred when fire broke out in the early hours of 1 November 1986 in a warehouse at a chemical factory in Basle, Switzerland, owned by Sandoz. The warehouse contained 1300 tonnes of chemicals, including pesticides, chemical dyes and organic compounds containing mercury. Among the 30 different agricultural chemicals were 25 tonnes of the insecticide parathion, 12 tonnes of the mercury based fungicide tillex, 10 tonnes of the insecticide fenitrothion, and 323 tonnes of the insecticide disulfoton. Hundreds of tonnes of other chemicals were washed into the Rhine when firehoses were played on the factory in an attempt to control the fire. The Rhine was rendered lifeless for 100–200 km as more pollutants were released in 2 hours than in a normal year. It is estimated that some 500 000 fish were killed outright; many of those that survived were contaminated with mercury. Although reports suggest that the Rhine is recovering, the continuing worry is that the chemicals may have permeated through the river bed into the underlying ground-waters. If this is so then water supplies in the Rhine basin may be polluted for years to come.

Within a month of the Sandoz fire, 12 major pollution incidents had been reported involving companies such as Ciba-Geigy (for the spillage of 100 gallons (450 litres) of atrazine into the Rhine, purportedly the day before the Sandoz accident) and BASF (leakage of 1100 kg of the herbicide 2,4-D from a plant near Ludwigshafen). However, there many lessons were undoubtedly learned from the Sandoz incident, which have subsequently led to action by both the industry and the fire authorities to prevent such an accident happening again.

STORAGE, TRANSPORT AND DISTRIBUTION

Pesticides need to be stored and transported at various stages of their progress between manufacturer and user: from manufacturer of active ingredient to formulator; from formulator to packer; packer to wholesaler; wholesaler to retail outlet; and retailer to user. Pesticides are transported by road, rail and water, and there have been a number of accidents recorded of pesticides in transit. The report of the Chairman of the Agriculture Committee into the effects of pesticides on human health[2] records recent examples of incidents in the UK, including the following:

1 Wildlife in the River Roding was destroyed along a 20 mile (32 km) stretch after a tanker carrying an insecticide on the M11 crashed near Abridge in 1985, spilling its load into the river.
2 Eighty barrels, each containing 440 pounds (240 kg) of dinoseb, were washed overboard from a cargo ship near the Dogger Bank in January 1984. By May, 67 barrels had been recovered, leaving 13 untraced in rich fishing grounds.

A well-publicized incident was the sinking of the *MV Parentis* in the English Channel on 13 March 1989. The cargo contained 5 tonnes of lindane, 1 tonne permethrin, and 600 kg cypermethrin. The principal concern was the fate of the container of lindane, which has still not been recovered. The manufacturers, Rhone-Poulenc, state that it is toxic to fish, but point out that the container is in three layers of packaging, and the chemical has low solubility at low temperatures. The persistence of lindane in the marine environment has been clearly demonstrated by the results of a survey of the levels in the North Sea carried out in the period 1986–88 on behalf of the West German Federal Ministry of Research and Technology. This work revealed the presence of relatively high levels of lindane in the

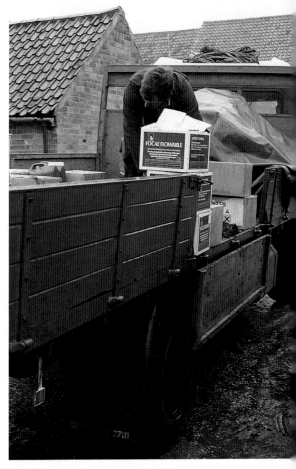

Pesticides must be transported safely

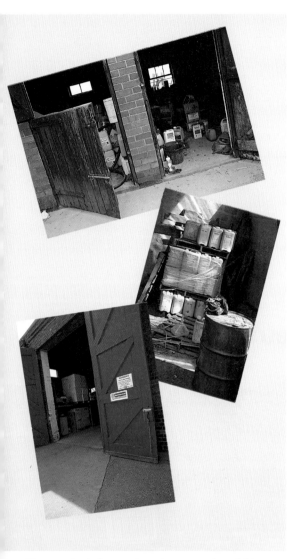

The standards for supply and storage of pesticides in the UK are set by the British Agrochemical Standards Inspection Scheme.

eastern England, the Netherlands, West Germany, Denmark and Norway. It also showed that concentrations of lindane in Hermit Crab (*Pagurus bernhardus*) were 'particularly high' in the southeastern North Sea, in those areas with the maximum concentration in sea water[77].

In the UK standards for the storage and supply of pesticides are set by the British Agrochemical Standards Inspection Scheme (BASIS). The siting of pesticide stores is subject to local authority regulations, while the transport of pesticides must conform to applicable national and international air, maritime, road and rail regulations for classification, packaging, labelling and transport of potentially dangerous substances. Once pesticides are delivered to a farm, the occupier has the responsibility to take all reasonable precautions to ensure that they are stored and transported so as to protect people and animals, and to safeguard the environment. Storage of pesticides is regulated by the Health and Safety at Work etc Act 1974, regulations made under COSHH, approved codes of practice, and by a Health and Safety Executive Guidance Note[78] which sets out the standards for storage on farms, in horticulture, by local authorities and so on. The following criteria should be met whatever the size of the store.

The store should be:

1 Suitably sited.
2 Large enough to hold the maximum capacity of pesticides likely to be kept at any one time.
3 Soundly constructed of fire-resistant materials.
4 Provided with suitable entrances and exits.
5 Capable of holding any spillages or leakages.
6 Dry and frost free.
7 Suitably lit and ventilated.
8 Properly equipped and organised.
9 Marked and secure against theft and vandalism.

The International Group of National Associations of Manufacturers of Agrochemical Products (GIFAP) has produced *Guidelines for the Safe Warehousing of Pesticides* and *Guidelines for Safe Transport of Pesticides*. The industry also issues its own standards, for example the *Safe Storage of Crop Protection Chemicals Standards* produced by ICI.

EXPORTS, IMPORTS AND THE AGROCHEMICAL MARKET

The 1970s were characterized by steady growth in agricultural production driven by strong demand, high commodity prices, high economic growth, and marked improvements in agricultural productivity. This agricultural boom fuelled a world-wide growth in the agrochemical industry too, averaging 6.3% per annum in real terms. Then in the early 1980s, world trade and economic growth slowed sharply. For the first time agricultural production in the developed world exceeded demand. The EEC became a net cereal exporter and the notorious European 'food mountains' grew as a result of a food policy based on subsidies. In 1983 a further brake was put on the agrochemical industry by the US Payment in Kind (PIK) programme, which led to a 2.9% real decline – the first ever recorded in the agrochemical market. Although growth recovered in 1984, it settled at a lower average rate of 1.1% per annum for the 4-year period 1984–87. Global sales in 1987 of about $20 billion represented another decline, only 4 years after the first in 1983[64].

In this environment, competition between companies has intensified. With reduced subsidies and lower farm incomes, farmers have become increasingly cost conscious. In addition, the expiry of patents on major products has generated more generic competition. As Table 3.5 shows, all of the top ten pesticides in the USA were introduced before 1976, and seven of them are now off-patent.

Technical solutions already exist for most plant protection problems, and market penetration by pesticide products is near maximum in developed countries. The agrochemical industry is therefore turning to new scientific developments, particularly in the area of biotechnology, and to emerging markets in developing countries. Rapid advances in biotechnology are leading to the development of novel microbial crop protection techniques, and to crop varieties that are resistant to pests. Because the research and development costs are prohibitively high for small biotechnology firms, several of these have been taken over by the larger agrochemical companies. If the current trend continues, both the pest control market and the seeds market will be controlled by a handful of companies by the end of the century.

However, according to industry analysts, biotechnology is unlikely to account for more than 5% of the total crop protection market by the turn of the century. Most new products will continue to be chemically based for the foreseeable future, with an emphasis on programmes to suppress the development of resistance, the production of very highly active products (with use rates measured in grams rather than kilograms per hectare) and new products to replace those withdrawn on environmental or safety grounds. The fastest growing market for these products is among developing countries like India and Brazil. The agrochemical industry forecasts growth rates of approximately 6% for both these countries for the period 1986–90[64].

Table 3.5
Top 10 US pesticides (1986). Patent status and launch dates

Product	Launch	Patent expired
Glyphosate	1972	No
Alachlor	1966	Yes
Metribuzin	1971	No
Carbaryl	1956	Yes
Chlorpyrifos	1965	Yes
Carbofuran	1967	Yes
Chlorothalonil	1963	Yes
Trifluralin	1963	Yes
Bentazon	1975	No
Dicamba	1965	Yes

Source: ICI Agrochemicals, in World Crop Protection Prospects: Demisting the Crystal Ball. The Bawden Memorial Lecture, Brighton Crop Protection Conference, 1988

Developing countries like Brazil represent a fast-growing market for pesticides products.

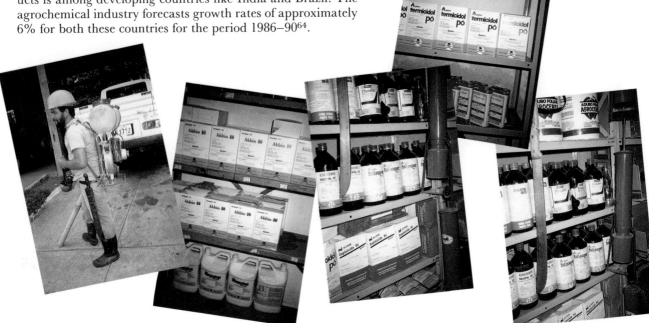

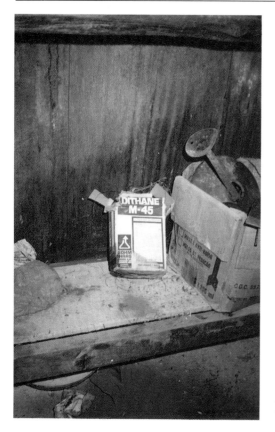

In recent years there has been concern expressed by bodies such as Oxfam and the Pesticides Action Network over the export of pesticides to Third World countries. The major concern is that pesticides that are banned in their country of origin, or that have restrictions on their use, are still exported to the developing world. According to an Oxfam report[41], approximately 30% of US pesticide exports in 1976 were of products whose use is prohibited in the USA. The FAO Code of Conduct on distribution and use of pesticides[79] (to which all members of the BAA are signatories) lays down clear standards for testing, distribution, promotion, product information, labelling and advertising. Major companies are also concerned with 'product stewardship', defined as 'responsible and ethical management of a product during its progress from invention to its ultimate use and beyond'[80]. However, even when products are exported in good faith there is little that can be done to prevent irresponsible handling by retailers and users. Pesticides are often packed in quantities that necessitate repackaging at the retail level with consequent dangers of exposure for the packer. The Oxfam report records incidents of repackaging in inappropriate containers with a lack of labelling for the final user. Such labels as there are may give incomplete safety information, often in a language other than that of the local community. Add to this the likelihood of high levels of illiteracy, lack of training, poor storage facilities, inadequate equipment and absence of effective legislative controls, and it is not surprising that there is a widespread incidence of pesticide poisoning in the Third World.

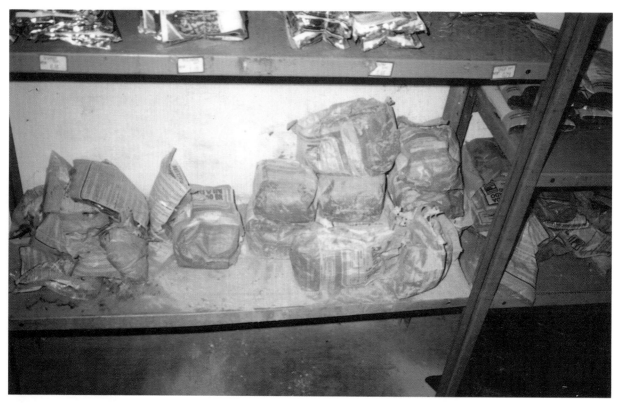

Storage conditions for pesticides in Third World countries may be poor.

Several international agencies including the European Commission and the FAO are considering ways in which the problem of industrialized countries exporting pesticides to nations with less well developed controls can be overcome. FAO has now further tightened up its Code of Conduct by naming on a 'red alert' list more than 50 pesticides and other chemicals that have been banned or severely restricted in five or more countries. Products on the list will be subject to the principles of Prior Informed Consent (PIC). PIC means that an exporting country intending to ship pesticides to an importing country should secure the importing country's specific consent before shipment. The consent should be informed, which means that the importing government should have full knowledge of the domestic regulatory status of the pesticide, including any bans or restrictions on its use[81]. The Netherlands has in place a voluntary PIC scheme, which has been commended by the European Council of Ministers. The United Nations Environment Programme (UNEP) agreed PIC procedures for chemicals in May 1989 and the FAO adopted PIC for pesticides on its red alert list in December 1989.

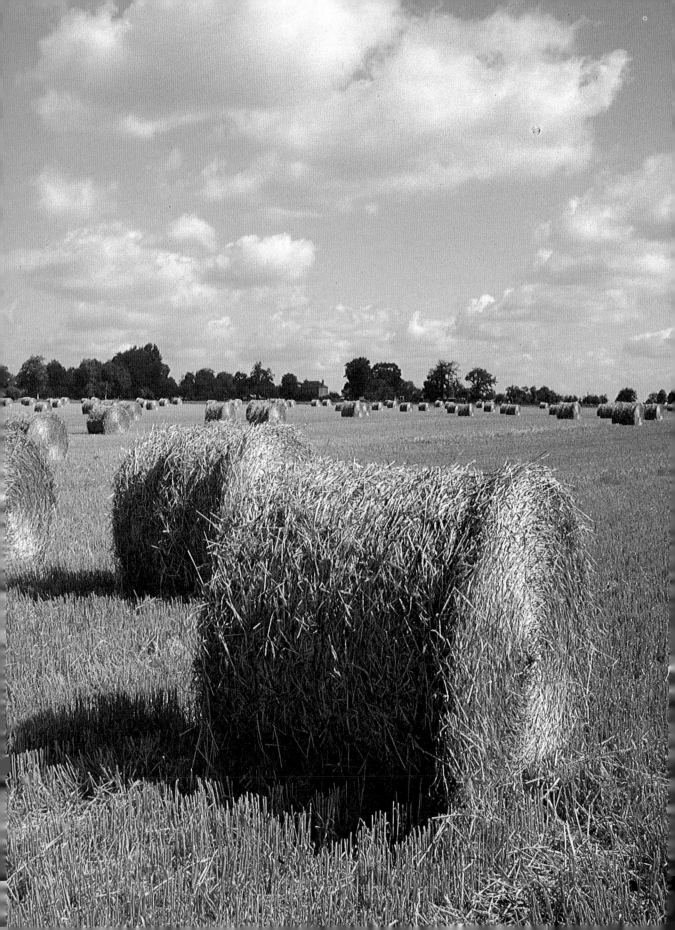

4 AREAS OF USE

Pesticides are sold, not only to professional users, but also to members of the public (in lower concentrations and smaller packages) for use in almost every area of our everyday lives – in agriculture, horticulture and forestry, in parks and recreational areas, in industry, on our pets, and in our homes and gardens[82]. Pesticides are not, of course, the only toxic substances available to the home gardener or do-it-yourself enthusiast. In any builder's merchant one can buy bleach, strong mineral acids, caustic soda, solvents, tars, cement, lead and so on. But the use of pesticides is particularly ubiquitous, and they are unusual in that they are designed to be active against biological systems. Many areas of use are obvious to the public at large – the spraying of agricultural crops, for example. The fact that pesticides are also used for the protection of carpets in storage, or that the anti-coagulant drug warfarin is the same chemical that was once used as rat poison, may be less well known by the lay person.

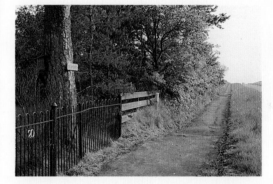

This tell-tale strip of yellowing grass bordering a public footpath was caused by the over-application of a path-clearing herbicide.

Pesticides are used in the following areas:

1 Agriculture.
2 Horticulture.
3 Fish farming.
4 Forestry.
5 Amenity use (parks, gardens, playing fields).
6 Fumigation and wood preservation.
7 Industrial pest control.
8 Manufactured products (wallpaper pastes, tile grout, paint, masonry treatment).
9 Homes and gardens.
10 Marine pest control (anti-fouling paints).
11 Aquatic pest control.
12 Food and commodity storage.
13 Animal husbandry (veterinary pesticides, animal medicines).
14 Public hygiene and pest control.
15 Human medicines.

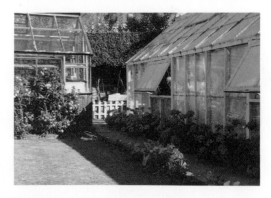

Pesticides are sold to the home gardener in lower concentrations and smaller packages.

AGRICULTURE AND HORTICULTURE

Consistent comparative figures on the level of pesticide use in agriculture are not easy to come by. However the figures, albeit for different years and different crops, make one thing very clear: a very high proportion of all crops are treated with pesticides. In England and Wales in 1974, 99.5% of the cereal crop was treated with pesticide, as was 98.4% of potatoes, sugar beet and field beans. In 1972 94% of vegetable crops were

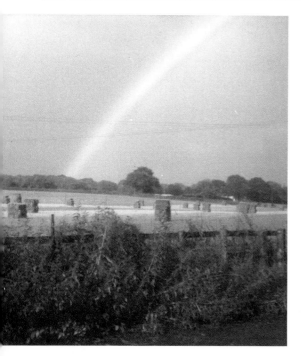

A very high proportion of all crops are treated with pesticides.

treated; in 1973 92% of orchards; in 1975 the entire hop crop; in 1975 99% of the soft fruit crop[3].

Most of these crops receive a series of pesticide applications. In England and Wales in 1977 42% of the cereal crop (1 347 918 hectares) received between four and six applications of pesticides. Five or more pesticides were used on 52% of winter wheat and 18 or more chemicals were used on 2% of the crop. Forty six per cent of other arable crops (218 960 hectares) received 4–6 applications of pesticide in the same year[3]. In 1977, 8% of winter wheat (81 984 hectares) received 10–14 applications of pesticide. Eighty three per cent of main crop potatoes were treated five or more times; 15% of this crop received 10–14 treatments. Five or more different chemicals were used on 36% of the main crop potato area planted. Eighty six per cent of seed potatoes (4807 hectares) received nine pesticide treatments per year[83]. General cereal crops regularly receive 5–8 applications per season, whereas for high value crops like fruit and vegetables 10–15 applications or more per season is normal.

However, the important question is not how frequently crops are sprayed, nor even how soon before harvesting, but the toxicity of the chemical and the amount of residue in the crop. In 1987 the California State Department of Food and Agriculture (CDFA) conducted an analysis of 13 400 samples taken from crops grown within and outside the state, and including some imported from outside the USA. The majority of crops sampled (over 80%) contained no detectable pesticide residues. These figures compare with recent residue surveys in the UK showing that 73% of food crops contained no detectable residues, and only 1% were actually over the Maximum Residue Level (MRL). The MRL is the level to be expected when the crop is sprayed according to the label, and is not a measure of safety. The measure of safety is given by the Acceptable Daily Intake (ADI), which is always below the MRL. The MRL is taken into account when setting the ADI.

The figures should also be compared with other assessments. For example, an independent survey undertaken in San Francisco[84] found that 44% of 71 fruit and vegetable samples contained residues of 19 different pesticides. In comparison, the state's own pesticide monitoring programme detected residues in only 7–20% of samples of the same crop types. An official report published in 1988[85] highlighted the State of California's inability to monitor satisfactorily pesticide residues in food. According to the report, the multi-residue analytical techniques used for residue testing in California fail to detect two-thirds of registered pesticides: there is no routine programme for testing processed foods and the system of food, tolerances and the monitoring techniques used in California are now seriously out of date.

There is also evidence of defects in the techniques used in the UK. The Residues Sub-Group of the Government's Research Consultative Committee on Cereals has reported that:

'In most cases the levels of residues of post-harvest fungicides and anti-oxidants used on some fruits have been measured in the skin only but recent work indicates that, in certain cases, pesticides penetrate into the flesh of the fruit. As a consequence it seems probable that residue levels are generally diluted, so that the concentrations in the flesh of the fruit may fall below levels which can be determined using current procedures. However, since the whole fruit is consumed, the total amount of pesticide in the fruit could be significantly more than that previously thought to be confined to the peel tissues. As a result, consumers may be exposed to higher dosages of the chemicals than has hitherto been suspected'[40].

The Sub-Group has also pointed out that about 80% of the UK apple and pear crop is held in long-term storage requiring some form of post-harvest chemical application. They stated that there is 'an urgent need to re-examine the reliability of existing data on residue levels'[40].

Most agricultural pesticides are purchased as liquid concentrate, diluted with water up to 200 times, and then applied as a spray. The diluted liquid is usually carried in a tank attached to the rear of a tractor, or towed behind, and a spray bar is used to distribute the pesticide. For most agricultural use, where large acreage has to be covered, the spray bar is directed downwards onto the crop. There should not be much pesticide drift and, so long as the driver remains within his or her enclosed cab, exposure should be minimal. The more serious potential for exposure arises when the farm worker is handling the concentrate[86,87].

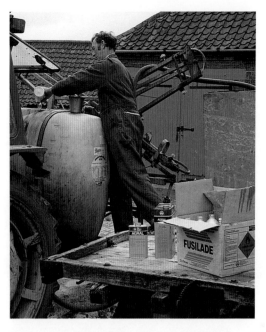

The farmer is at particular risk of exposure to concentrated pesticide during the preparation of diluted mixture for application.

The use of a tractor mounted spray boom enables crop spraying to be carried out over a large area.

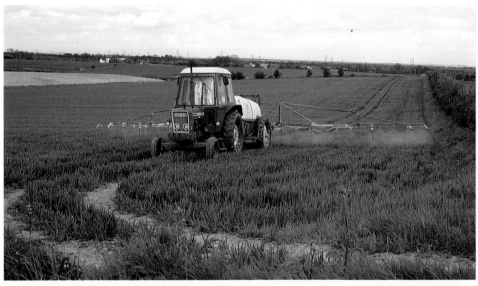

The spraying of fruit trees in orchards can be a more hazardous operation when spray is directed upwards under high pressure to reach fruit at the top. Unless the tractor has a well-sealed cab the driver is much more likely to become contaminated than when using a downwards directed spray. Currently apple and pear trees are treated several times in a season to combat two types of enemy: pests such as the codlin-moth and the red spider mite, and a range of fungal diseases of which the most persistent are mildew and scab[88]. The status of the apple as an emblem of good health has undoubtedly fuelled the controversy surrounding the presence of pesticide residues (in particular Alar) on the fruit.

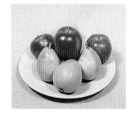

Pesticide residue may be contained in both the peel and flesh of fruit.

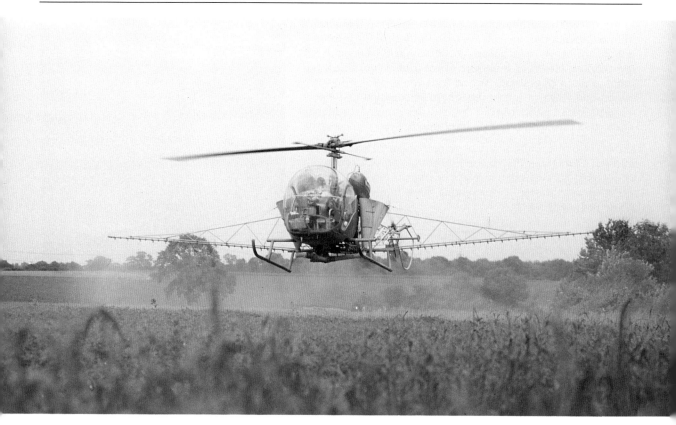

There is greater potential for accidental exposure to pesticide spray during aerial application than from ground-based application.

Aerial crop spraying accounts for only 2% or less of all pesticide applications (less than 1% of pesticide ingredients by weight), but it is a focus of public concern. Misuse has a greater potential for accidental contamination of local inhabitants, passers-by, schoolchildren, domestic gardens and watercourses than ground-based application of pesticides. Aerial spraying was developed in the 1920s when lead arsenate was used to control the catalpa sphinx in the USA. Crop dusting became an important source of work for pilots who had flown in the world wars, and its use spread rapidly in the vast grain-growing regions of the USA. Aerial application has also played an important role in many disease control programmes in the Third World, including action against malaria, bilharzia, and other human diseases, and for spraying against locust swarms to improve agricultural production[89].

In Britain, aerial spraying has never been as widely used as in the USA, but it did experience a steady rise during the 1970s. In 1977 628000 hectares were sprayed by 114 aircraft. By 1987, as recession and falling agricultural quotas started to hit farming, the number of hectares treated by aerial applications had halved (Figure 4.1).

An additional factor in the reduction of aerial spraying may have been a reduction in the numbers of types of pests (for example, aphids) against which aerial spraying is targeted.

Figures from the recent Agricultural Development and Advisory Service (ADAS) survey report on aerial pesticide applications in Great Britain[90] show the areas of the country where aerial spraying is most likely to be encountered and the types of pesticide most commonly applied by air (Figure 4.2).

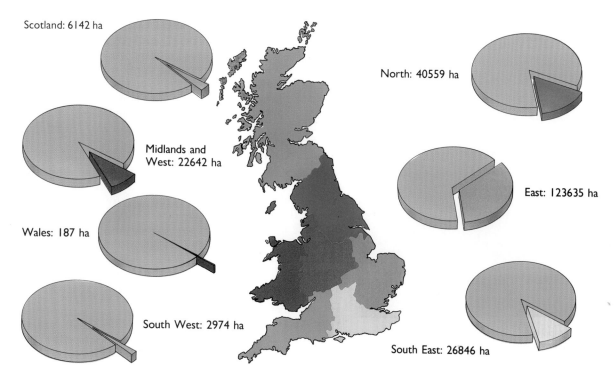

Scotland: 6142 ha

North: 40559 ha

Midlands and West: 22642 ha

East: 123635 ha

Wales: 187 ha

South West: 2974 ha

South East: 26846 ha

Figure 4.1
Distribution of treated areas in Great Britain and proportions of total area treated from the air.

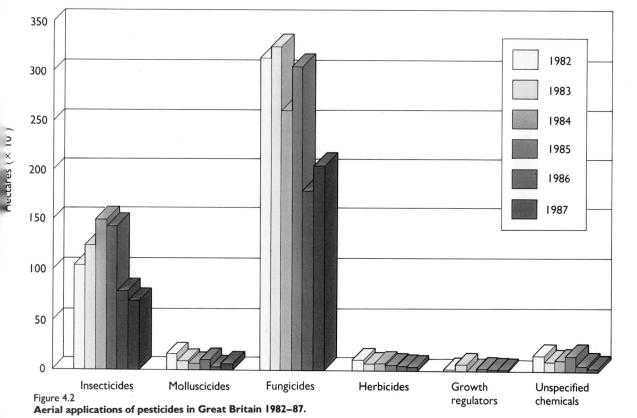

Figure 4.2
Aerial applications of pesticides in Great Britain 1982–87.

Returns of pesticide applications made by aerial contractors in 1987, and reported in the ADAS survey, show the largest areas of treatment were on oilseed rape, potatoes, peas, beans and cereals. The most extensively applied chemical groups were fungicides, followed by organophosphorus and carbamate insecticides. Fifty-one per cent of applications were made by helicopter and the remainder by fixed wing aircraft[90].

Aerial spraying inevitably causes a much greater drift than pesticide spraying from a tractor mounted boom. A survey by the US Environmental Protection Agency in 1975[91] showed that between 10% and 60% of spray droplets drifted more than 1000 ft (approximately 300 m) from the target. However, because of the very small size of droplets produced in pesticide spraying, the aggregate volume of pesticide in spray drift is very small. In the UK, Civil Aviation Authority (CAA) regulations specify that an aircraft can pass within 200 ft (61 m) of a dwelling house. In Germany the distance is 50–100 m, in Holland 110–150 m, in Denmark 300 m and in Belgium 200 m. In Eire (15 m) it is less than in the UK[92]. Research by the Soil Association into spray drift[89] has identified five main types of aerial spraying incident (all of which are illegal acts):

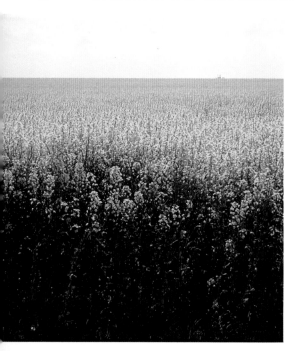

Oilseed rape is one of the main crops treated by aerial spraying.

1 Overshooting the target area and spraying surrounding gardens, houses, roads and villages. This usually occurs because the pilot tries to spray right up to the edge of the field, or fails to switch off the spray while turning, or because of wind drift.
2 Applying pesticide in unsuitable weather conditions, usually during high winds.
3 Flying too low or too near houses, in contravention of the CAA regulations.
4 Spraying the incorrect area altogether through failure to identify the target field.
5 Accidents involving aircraft used for spraying, including colliding with power lines and other aircraft. Aerial spraying is a high risk activity because of the continuous low level flying.

Pilot fatigue and error will inevitably produce a high level of casualties. There is also the possibility of pilots being poisoned by their own spray. A survey in Canada found that out of 167 crashes of crop spraying aircraft, 15 were due to the toxic effects of pesticides on the pilot[93].

A report by the CAA, covering the period 1976-87, lists 139 accidents in the UK involving helicopters (75 cases) or fixed-wing aircraft (64 cases) which were engaged in crop spraying. Five of these accidents caused fatalities[94].

Reports by the Soil Association[89], Friends of the Earth[92], and Health and Safety Executive (HSE) annual reports all contain a series of case studies of aerial spraying incidents. Pesticide incidents involving allegations of ill health or misuse are now investigated by HM Agricultural Inspectorate Division of the HSE. The Pesticides Incidents Appraisal Panel (PIAP), which includes representatives from HM Agricultural Inspectorate, Department of Health Toxicology Section, Employment Medical Advisory Service, and National Poisons Information Units, considers all investigated incidents and classifies them as confirmed, likely, unlikely or not yet confirmed. In 1988 160

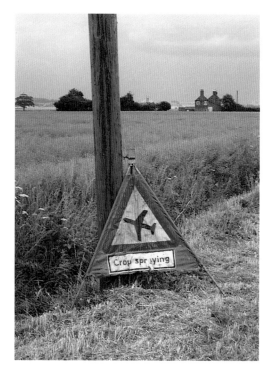

Warning sign.

pesticide incidents were investigated, a slight increase on the 1987 total of 145. Of these, 12 in 1988 and 44 in 1987 related to aerial spraying incidents where prosecution took place by the HSE[95]. As is the way with many complaints, the reports are sometimes vague ('it was pretty windy') and emotive (members of the public were 'cowering' beneath a low flying spraying helicopter), but there are substantiated cases of spraying without prior notification and of drift onto nearby individuals and property. It is important to remember that the number of incidents that do occur are small compared with the amount of pesticide used throughout the UK. Millions of pesticide packs are opened every year; in 1988 these resulted in only 160 investigated cases, not all of which related to aerial spraying.

DEVELOPING TRAINING TECHNIQUES

The best method of training workers in the method of use and disposal would be the development of engineering controls which prevent contact between chemical and user. This is a requirement under the COSHH Regulations 1988.

The research, testing and development of spraying systems and other application techniques, which are safer to the operator and environment should be given priority. Improvements in application efficiency and safety have a direct spin-off in terms of protecting the public and environmental health, and in reducing the amount of residues in food and water.

Application hazards should be controlled by the use of technical and engineering controls and not, as industry has done in the past, by over-reliance on personal protective equipment as the main means of operator protection. This means everything from better design of containers and improved design of knapsack sprayers to the fitting of pesticide filters in cabs, sealed mixing and filling systems, through to safer disposal equipment.

Sprayer technology has, in general, lagged behind the development and introduction of the pesticides it is used to apply. Hydraulic spraying – the most commonly used type – by its very nature creates spray drift, which is a serious problem for operators and wildlife, as well as damaging crops and polluting water courses. More research and development of improved/alternative spraying systems such as CDA/ULV and electrostatic spraying is needed. Poor calibration and setting up of spraying and application equipment is another problem area and one that poses risk to the consumer as crops can be easily overlooked, leading to excessive residue levels in harvested and stored produce. Similarly, improved pesticide mixing, filling and disposal systems need developing. Operators are particularly at risk when handling pesticide concentrate during mixing and filling operations and sealed systems need to be developed.

Pesticide disposal is a grey area. Lack of safe disposal techniques and equipment for waste, diluted pesticide concentrate and for empty pesticide containers threatens human and environmental health. Disposing of waste pesticide on farm landfill and containers by landfill/burning is no longer seen as satisfactory in terms of protecting wildlife and the environment.

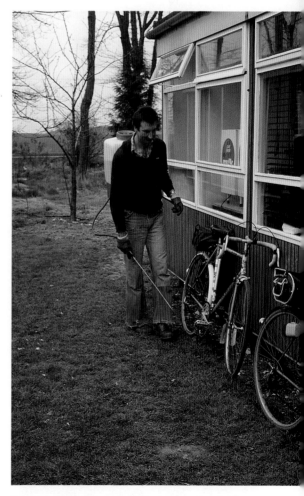

Because of the close proximity to the spray during knapsack spraying, protective clothing should be worn.

Increasing attention is being paid by government and industry and users to the problem of safe disposal. There is increasing pressure on pesticide manufacturers, particulary from the farming community, to implement 'reverse chain' disposal, whereby the manufacturers/suppliers would have an obligation to help dispose of revoked pesticide (where the approval is withdrawn or lapses), unwanted pesticide concentrate, as well as washed, empty containers.

LIVESTOCK AND FISH FARMING

Pesticides are also widely used in the livestock production area of agriculture. These may be as 'animal medicines' when applied directly to the animal as in sheep dips, warble fly dressings, and lice/mange treatments, or as 'veterinary pesticides' when used in livestock houses for the control of flies or other insects. Pesticides used in livestock management

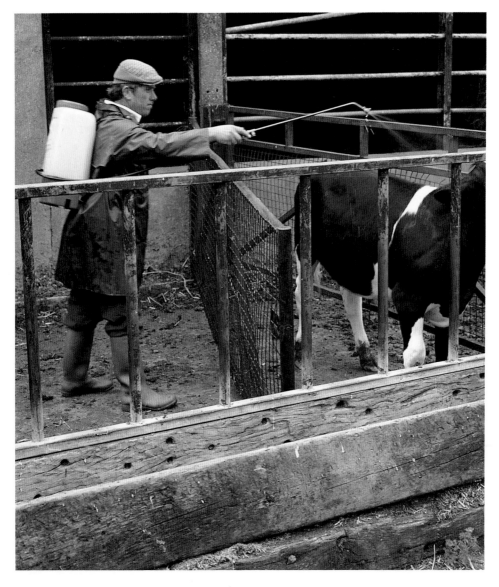

Pesticides are used widely in livedstock productions.

include carbaryl (a carbamate insecticide used as a veterinary pesticide to control fleas, lice and so on); dioxathion (an organophosphorus insecticide used to control parasites like ticks); ethion (a broad spectrum insecticide used on cattle); malathion (an organophosphorus insecticide used to control animal parasites, flies, lice, and insects in homes and agricultural buildings); and toxaphene and trichlorofon (insecticides used for livestock pest control). The insecticide lindane, commonly found in wood preservatives in the UK although banned or restricted in some other countries, is also found in livestock products, specifically ectoparasite powders[96].

An important growth area for pesticide use is fish farming. Production of fish rose from 2500 tonnes in 1984 to 19 500 tonnes in 1988, and this rapid increase is set to continue. The Department of Agriculture and Fisheries for Scotland predicted that it would reach 54 000 tonnes by the early 1990s. Scientists, however, know very little about the effects salmon farms will have on the environment, especially the use of chemicals. The synthetic colouring, canthaxanthin (E161g), banned in the USA, is added to the diet as it makes the flesh of the fish pink like that of wild salmon, rather than 'hatchery grey'. The fish and their sea cages are kept clean with calcium oxide, chlorine, sodium hydroxide and iodophors (a solution of iodine). Disease is kept at bay with formaldehyde, malachite green and four common antibiotics.

Pesticides are used in fish farming for protection against diseases and infestation.

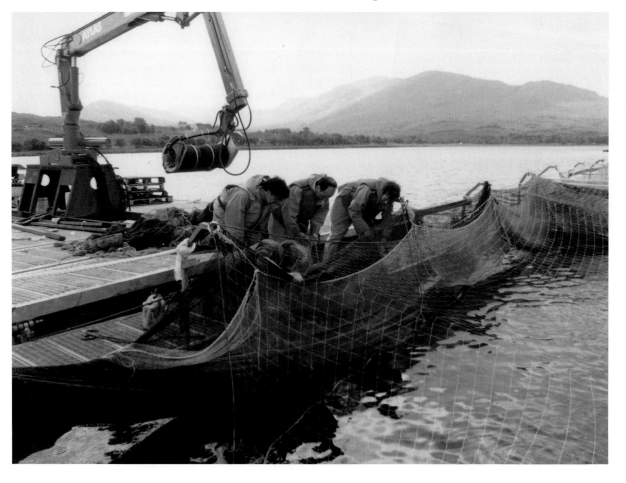

One chemical giving some cause for concern is dichlorvos (commercial names Nuvan and Aquagard), which salmon farmers insist is the only effective weapon against infestations of the parasitic salmon louse *Lepeophtheirus salmonis*. Dichlorvos, is an organophosphorus insecticide used in many settings, for example to control pests on glasshouse crops, mushrooms, fruit and vegetables, and to control flies and fleas on animals. In aquatic environments it is also toxic to crabs, shrimps, lobsters and mussels[83], although at the approved dosage levels there is no substantive evidence of toxicity to sea fauna[97]. HSE Agricultural Inspectors in Scotland, following the introduction of the Food and Environment Protection Act legislation in 1985, discovered dichlorvos was being used illegally to kill the salmon louse. At the time it was not approved for use for salmon, nor by fish farm workers for this purpose. The Government response was to reclassify dichlorvos as an 'animal medicine', effectively removing it from health and safety legislation. In Norway the sea wrasse is being used as a 'cleaner fish' to keep salmon free from lice. Evidence suggests that, although it has been used successfully only on an experimental basis, it provides the possibility of a non-toxic, biological alternative to dichlorvos which merits further investigation[97].

FORESTRY

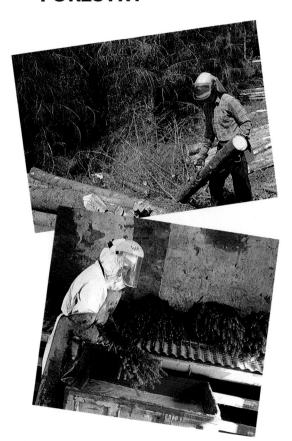

Pesticides are used widely at all stages of forest management. Forest nurseries and plantations are treated with several preparations to control weeds before planting and while the saplings are still young. The trees themselves receive overall spray treatment, as well as more localized band and spot treatment. Lindane and permethrin are extensively used for the treatment of forestry plantations, and there is also use of urea and peniophora to treat tree stumps after felling. Rodents are controlled using gassing tablets, powders and bait poisons[98].

Coniferous trees planted on clear felled land are highly susceptible to attack from the *Hylobius* abietis and *Hyalastes* species of beetle. In some cases there has been 100% damage to a newly planted forest. As beetle attacks cannot be accurately forecast the Forestry Commission now treats all coniferous trees by dipping young plants into a tank of lindane or permethrin, and then placing them on benches to drain. The plants are then heeled into the ground until they are moved to the forest for planting. Unless careful precautions are taken forestry workers are at risk from contamination when dipping or when planting the treated trees. Over the last 5 years the Forestry Commission has, in conjunction with ICI, been developing an improved system using an electrostatic sprayer to apply a measured amount of pesticide to each tree. The equipment should have significant advantages over the old system in terms of user safety and plant handling[99]. Similar attention does not yet seem to have been devoted to the risks attached to the use of handheld ultra-low volume sprayers in forestry. The use of such equipment also exposes the worker to a substantial risk of contamination, and necessitates the wearing of considerable protective clothing[83].

Pesticides are used at all stages of forest managment.

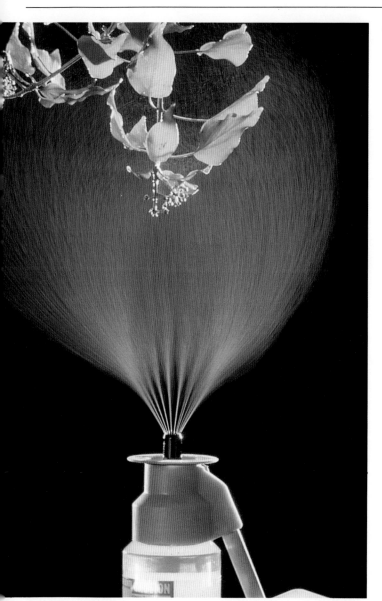

An electrostatic sprayer.

PUBLIC AMENITIES AND UTILITIES

Local authorities are important pesticide users in public parks and gardens, playing fields, sports facilities, on town pavements, around housing estates and other council properties. Pesticides are used to maintain turf quality at golf clubs, tennis clubs, bowling greens and cricket grounds. Highway authorities regularly spray roadside verges and pavements, roundabouts and other areas. British Rail contractors spray thousands of kilos of herbicides, largely atrazine and simazine, onto railway lines and embankments every year. These pesticides are commonly found in ground-water in the UK[83]. Railway lines are sprayed to stop weeds and small trees interfering with the safe operation of the railway. The ballast bed of railway lines must remain flexible and spongy, since this plays a vital part in the suspension of trains. If weeds are allowed to grow, their roots bind the ballast together, leaving it rigid. The use of pesticides on railway lines is an example of the balance of risks and benefits.

Other pesticides used in public areas are growth regulators and aquatic herbicides[100]. Growth regulators are used to reduce growth on roadside verges, embankments, airfields, and in cemeteries.

They also limit the size of hedges, ornamental and bedding plants, and keep in check the growth of grass on areas such as golf and bowling greens. Active ingredients include maleic hydrazide and mefluidide. Maleic hydrazide is also used in aquatic weed control in addition to a number of other herbicides. Because of the dangers to the water supply there are strict standards for the use of aquatic herbicides. The only herbicides that can be used for weed control in or near water are asulam, fosamine ammonium, 2,4-D amine, maleic hydrazide and glyphosphate for the control of bracken, shrubs, bushes, grasses, and broad leaved plants on banks; and diquat, dichlobenil and terbutryne for control of submerged and floating plants and algae.

FUMIGATION AND WOOD PRESERVATION

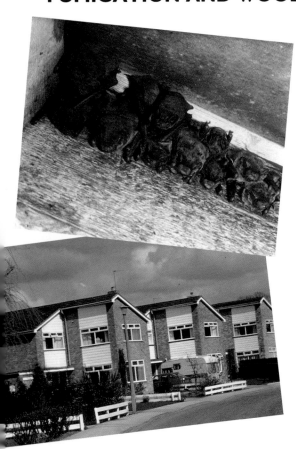

Many chemicals used in the treatment of new housing materials are toxic to bats which are a protected species.

Pesticides are present in wood preservatives used to kill the fungi and wood-boring insects which can attack exposed or neglected timber. For its first 100 years the timber preservation industry was confined almost entirely to the pre-treatment of wood for outside use. Railway sleepers, telegraph poles and marine piles were impregnated with metal salts, creosote and arsenic. Only in the last 40 years – with the mass production of synthetic insecticides, fungicides, and organic solvents – has wood preservation come indoors, with the spraying and fumigation of the places where people live and work. Timber preservation is now big business, with the industry divided into two sectors. The pre-treatment sector supplies pesticide-treated timbers for houses, buildings and outdoor use, including underwater timbers and boats. The remedial treatment sector has grown, as more building societies are now routinely demanding guarantees of timber treatment. Modern building practice, in particular the use of soft sapwoods, often provides the conditions that make the use of wood preservatives necessary. Today hundreds of wood preservation companies place around 100 tonnes of chemicals a year into homes and other buildings in over 150 000 treatments.

Chemicals used in timber treatment include the widely used creosote, which is banned in the USA for all but professional use; dieldrin, an insecticide only permitted for pre-treatment and approved in the USA only for termite control; PCP (pentachlorophenol), a fungicide used for pre-treatment and remedial work; TBTO (tributyltin oxide), a fungicide used in pre-treatment, remedial work, and DIY; and lindane, an insecticide used in pre-treatment and remedial work, and common in DIY products. Less hazardous pesticides, approved by the Nature Conservancy Council for use on bat roosts, include permethrin and boron compounds. Fumigants are used in a variety of situations, including the sterilization of grain houses to prevent insects and mould growth, in glasshouses, food stores and warehouses. Fumigation operations are controlled by law and there is an HSE Approved Code of Practice on Pesticide Fumigants, including ethylene oxide, hydrogen cyanide, methyl bromide, and phosphine.

TBTO was withdrawn from use as an anti-fouling paint on marine timbers and boats after it was shown to cause sexual deformities in dog whelks. The fungicide folpet, which was once widely used in anti-fouling paints, is no longer approved for use in the UK. The focus of concern has now shifted to lindane. Lindane (gamma hexachlorocyclohexane) has been in use since the 1930s, and currently over 80 companies produce between them more than 300 wood preservatives containing lindane as an active ingredient. The controversy surrounding wood preservatives received impetus and publicity from media coverage in 1987 and 1988, which reported the results of a survey of construction workers by the Union of Construction, Allied Trades and Technicians[101]. In the survey, allegations were made of illnesses following exposure of workers to wood preservatives.

There followed further allegations of illness among factory workers who produced the chemicals, of schoolchildren and staff in treated schools, and householders whose homes had been treated. A case widely reported in the press was that of a 13-year-old boy who developed aplastic anaemia after his home was treated with such products. As the commonest cause of aplastic anaemia in teenagers is a serious side effect of the relatively common childhood infection, hepatitis A (yellow jaundice), it is not possible to attribute causation in this case. Overall the evidence of the effects on health of wood preservatives is anecdotal and difficult to verify. A detailed collection of cases is given in a book from the London Hazards Centre called *Toxic Treatments*[102]. The London Hazards Centre is also creating a searchable database containing details of all known cases of illness apparently connected with exposure to wood preservatives. At the end of 1988 the Advisory Committee on Pesticides ordered a review of lindane; TBTO went under review in July 1987. No association between lindane and aplastic anaemia was found by the Advisory Committee on Pesticides.

MANUFACTURED PRODUCTS

Pesticides are present in a number of manufactured products. Examples include DIY products (wood preservatives, damp proofing treatments and wallpaper pastes), veterinary and human medicines, and marine anti-fouling paints. The persistent organochlorine insecticide aldrin is used to treat electric cables. In the USA aldrin/dieldrin has been judged carcinogenic for many years; in the UK it has been used extensively by Cornish daffodil growers but this use is now banned following the discovery of high levels of the chemical in eels in the Newlyn River, near Penzance.

In the home, many new carpets are treated with permethrin (an insecticide), with the trade name Mitin FF (an organochlorine compound, which is also used as a wood preserva-

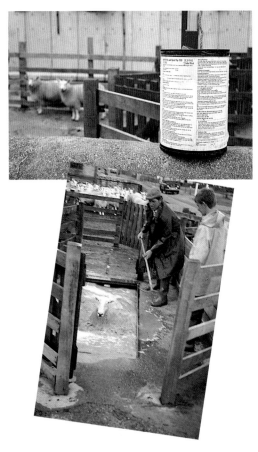

Lanolin (wool fat) which is present in some ointments may be contaminated with pesticides from sheep dips.

tive). Workers regularly handling permethrin have suffered from skin irritation and headaches, but according to the wool industry the pesticides bind to the wool fibres so only tiny amounts come into contact with the skin. Dichlorophen, a contact herbicide, fungicide and bactericide, is also used to protect fabrics against moulds.

In human medicine, warfarin, a rodenticide, is an anti-coagulant, widely used to prevent blood clots. Insecticides such as carbaryl, lindane and malathion are used in shampoos for control of human head lice and scabies, as well as pet delousing products. Recent studies in Australia[103] and in the USA[104] have drawn attention to the pesticide content of lanolin used as both an absorbent ointment and an ointment base. In the USA, as in the UK, lanolin is obtained from both domestic and foreign sheep, and it seems that pesticides contaminate the lanolin (wool fat) via sheep dips. Sheep dip preparations are formulated to resist rain and hence they can persist in lanolin long after the wool has been washed. Lanolin is used in a number of pharmaceutical and cosmetic preparations, but there has been some concern about the use of anhydrous lanolin to treat sore, cracked nipples in breast-feeding mothers. Analyses by the US Food and Drug Administration (FDA) and the Environmental Protection Agency (EPA) found chlorpyrifos, dieldrin, lindane, and DDE in lanolin samples. Pesticide levels in these samples were significantly higher than in lanolin products analysed by the FDA a few years ago. Although the levels were not high enough to present an immediate toxic hazard, safe quantities were hard to define. A letter in the *Journal of the American Medical Association (JAMA)*[104], suggested, 'it seems unnecessary knowingly to apply toxic chemicals directly to the skin and, in the case of breast-fed infants, to directly feed a toxin to a baby via lanolin on the nipple.' Despite this note of caution the risk to breast-feeding infants must be tiny.

HOMES AND GARDENS

As we have seen, pesticides are present in our homes, in our garages and DIY cupboards, in the bathroom cabinet and on the dressing table, and in the carpets on our floor. We apply pesticides to our houseplants, spray them on flies and mosquitoes, hang them up as fly killing strips, put them on our pets, leave them around to kill mice and rats, and use them to treat woodworm. When we buy shampoos and shelf paper, mattresses and shower curtains, we may unwittingly be bringing pesticides into our homes. But it is when we step out into the garden that we come into contact with the greatest range of domestic pesticides. According to the Soil Association, British gardeners spend about £15 million in shops and garden centres every year, buying a million or so kilos of sprays, dusts and aerosols, choosing from a range of 500 brand name products[105]. The most recent figures from the British Agrochemicals Association (BAA)[106] show that over the period 1982–88 sales in £m of garden herbicides increased by 20.9% and garden insecticides by 35.1%. Only garden and household fungicides fell, by 11.1%. Garden centres cater for every imaginable garden problem, selling herbicides, insecticides, acaricides, molluscicides, fungicides and weedkiller mixes, down to washes to remove moss from stones. Again according to the Soil Association, gardeners use a kilo of formulated product per acre of garden every year[105]. However, a typical concentration of active ingredient in a product is only 5%, with 95% made up of inerts, carriers and so on. Domestic garden pesticides are of a lower toxicity than those produced for the professional market, so that home users do not require protective clothing.

A survey carried out by the Soil Association in 1986[105] examined published health and safety data from Europe and North America relating specifically to pesticides sold for home garden use in the UK. The survey suggested that a large number had 'known or suspected adverse effects on health'. These included 38 chemicals described as irritating to the eyes, skin or respiratory tract; 25 with known or suspected carcinogenic effects in animals; and 29 known or suspected mutagens or teratogens (again in animals at high doses). Other formulations are harmful to animals, including birds, butterflies, bees, pets and garden fish. Some require a harvest interval between their application and eating the crop, to allow the chemical to break down into less harmful residues. Several are acute poisons which can kill if taken accidentally, for example by a child.

Many popular gardening books recommend a veritable arsenal of garden pesticides. By far the most successful have been the cheaply priced and cleverly designed *Be Your Own Garden Expert Series*, written by Dr D. G. Hessayon. These have sold over 30 million copies since the Second World War and can be found on the shelves of most amateur gardeners. The author is the Chairman of Pan Britannica Industries (PBI), a major pesticide manufacturer, and the books have been accused by some, including the Soil Association, of being 'essentially glossy sales brochures for PBI products'[105]. An examination of the booklets devoted to pest control, *Be Your Own Vegetable Doctor* and *Be Your Own Garden Doctor*, shows that pesticides marketed by ICI, Fisons, Secto and others are listed alongside PBI products. There is also useful advice on prevention, as well as treatment by more traditional means (for example, chopping up cutworms with a hoe), but there is no doubt that the *Garden Expert* books and most others on sale present the view that spraying with a range of pesticides is the norm in the domestic garden. However, with the setting up of centres such as the Henry Doubleday Research Association's National Centre for Organic Gardening at Ryton-on-Dunsmore, Coventry, gardeners may obtain advice on all forms of preventative measures such as intercropping, and on organic gardening.

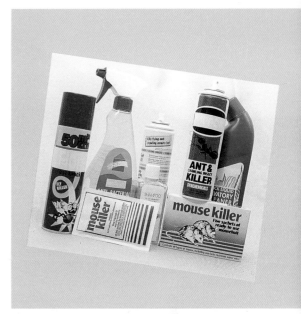

Examples of some household products containing pesticides.

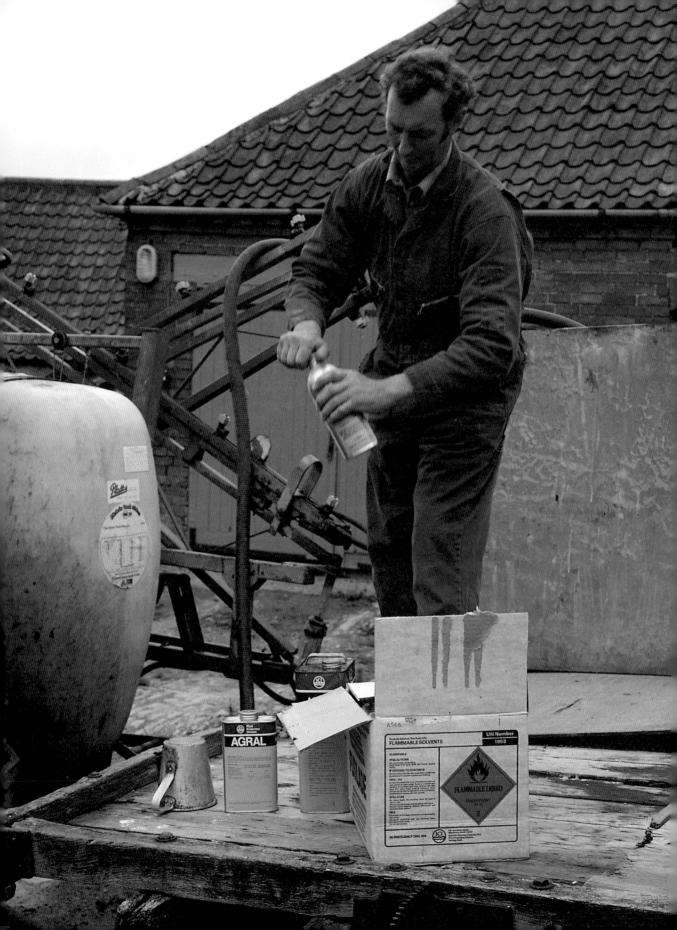

5 EFFECTS ON INDIVIDUAL HEALTH

SHORT-TERM HEALTH EFFECTS

Most of the evidence on the adverse health effects of pesticides relates to acute exposure and acute poisoning. This almost certainly reflects the much greater likelihood of identifying the probable cause when the effects on health follow very soon after a noticeable pesticide exposure incident. Moreover, many pesticides and their solvents have an unpleasant smell which heightens awareness of exposure. Evidence of this was supplied to the House of Commons Select Committee[2] by the Medical Research Council (MRC), who stated that only four deaths from accidental pesticide poisoning occurred in Great Britain in 1980, while there were 798 deaths from accidental poisonings by other chemicals. Indeed the number of recorded deaths from accidental pesticide poisoning may be even fewer. Drawing on Health and Safety Executive (HSE) figures, Goulding[107] gives one death in 1978, two in 1979 and one in 1980. In the 1940s highly toxic materials such as arsenic, nicotine and sulphuric acid were used as pesticides, and some of the older organophosphorus compounds and herbicides such as DNOC were also extremely toxic. These have now largely been replaced by pesticides with a much more specific activity.

In terms of acute toxicity, the more recently introduced insecticides are certainly less toxic and persistent than the older organochlorine, organophosphorus and carbamate insecticides. Nevertheless, there are still incidents of acute poisoning from a wide range of pesticides following their accidental or deliberate ingestion, or skin contamination following careless handling of pesticide concentrates. Acute reactions usually occur while the chemical is being used or shortly afterwards. Most acute reactions last only a short time, and the majority of victims recover completely, without long-term complications. However, a few people may suffer permanent damage of some kind.

How Pesticides Enter the Body

If we are to understand the effects of acute pesticide poisoning, we need to know how pesticides can enter the body. Figure 5.1 shows the principal modes of chemical entry and exit, to and from a simplified human body.

The three routes of entry for pesticides, or any other chemical, are the skin, the lungs and the gut[108]. The gut and lungs have surface areas much greater than might at first be apparent. In the gut this is due to the villi, finger-like protrusions into the gut cavity. In the lungs it is due to the many fine alveoli at the ends of the airways. These increase the area of contact enormously and help the passage of chemicals into the blood. The

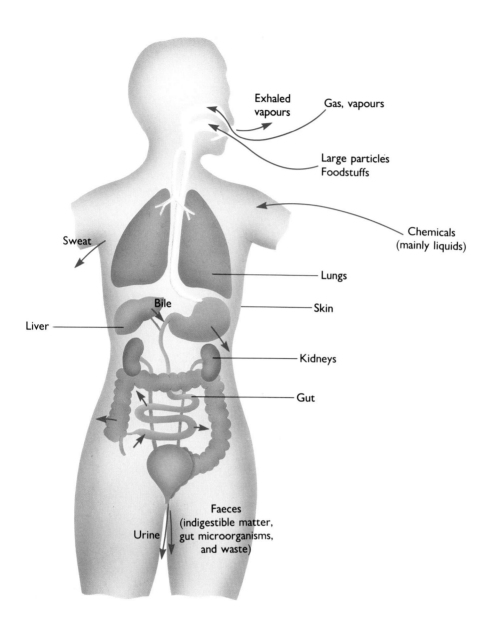

Exhaled vapours

Gas, vapours

Large particles
Foodstuffs

Chemicals
(mainly liquids)

Sweat

Lungs

Bile

Skin

Liver

Kidneys

Gut

Faeces
(indigestible matter,
gut microorganisms,
and waste)

Urine

Figure 5.1
Chemicals enter the body by ingestion inhalation and absorption through the gut, lungs and skin. Once absorbed, chemicals are metabolised or 'broken down' and eventually excreted through exhaled vapours, sweat, urine and faeces.

skin of a human adult has a superficial surface area of approximately 1.8 m^2, but folds and minute irregularities increase this area[108].

Absorption through the skin

Contamination of the skin with subsequent absorption of a pesticide is undoubtedly the major form of accidental acute exposure. Pesticides vary in their ability to permeate the skin. This depends, in part, on the nature of the formulation. Liquid formulations, especially those containing some organic solvents, may permeate more rapidly than, for instance, solid or aqueous-based products. However, extensive contamination of the skin may in certain cases have serious consequences within a few minutes.

The permeability of the skin is susceptible to alteration by chemicals, so that a substance that does not enter quickly by itself may be helped in by a second chemical which causes damage to the skin. Once chemicals enter the dermis and reach the skin capillaries they are rapidly transferred around the body in the blood stream. Dermatitis, both irritant and allergic, may be caused by certain chemicals, including pesticides[108]. It can also be caused by fruit and vegetables, shellfish, plants and animals, and many other natural materials.

Inhalation

The respiratory tract provides a very efficient surface for the absorption of substances, whether they are in the form of vapours, particles or droplets. Vapours are invisible free molecules in the air (for instance, air is 20–100% saturated with water vapour). Smoke and fume consists of very small particles, with a diameter of less than 1 µm. They often remain suspended in the air forever, because they are too light to be significantly attracted by gravity, and the movement of the air keeps them aloft. Droplets are generally defined as being greater than 200 µm, and these fall to the ground relatively quickly (for example, raindrops). In between, at diameters of 1 µm to 200 µm, is the range that is generally found in spraying. The respiratory system is a very efficient filter for the removal of aerosols, and particles larger than about 30 µm would not get beyond the nose or naso-pharynx. Particles down to about 7 µm will generally impact on the bronchi, and only those particles less than about 7 µm actually enter the alveoli.

The quantity of a chemical inhaled will vary with the frequency and depth of breathing. Frequency can vary from about 14 breaths a minute for an adult at rest to 25 or 30 for someone doing hard work. The volume of air taken in per breath (tidal volume) can vary from 0.5 litre (at rest) to 3–5 litres (working). Vapour that is very soluble in water will probably never reach the lungs, but be absorbed largely through the damp walls in the nose and the bronchial tree. Chemicals that are not readily soluble in water will be absorbed less rapidly in the lungs.

Ingestion

The gut is a very efficient mechanism for absorption of many materials; it can be also quite an efficient barrier to others. Although most chemicals only remain in the mouth for a short time, compounds can be absorbed through the mucous membranes. It is important that this be considered in the case of accidental poisoning because it is possible, even if the toxic substance taken into the mouth is spat out, that significant absorption may already have taken place before any of the material is swallowed[108]. If the chemical is not voided from the mouth, it enters the gastrointestinal tract. No significant absorption occurs in the oesophagus, and the toxicant passes on to enter the stomach.

Chemicals that are soluble in both water and fats are usually taken up more quickly than those that show solubility in only one or the other. In addition, the proportion of a chemical that is absorbed by the gut depends on the movements of the gut and the rate of passage of foodstuffs through it. At the lower end of the gut the chemicals taken in may be modified by intestinal micro-organisms to less toxic materials.

As chemicals are broken down they tend to become less toxic, as energy is extracted and molecules are broken down in the metabolic process. However, some pesticide degradation products are more toxic than the parent compound. For instance, the EBDC fungicides break down, especially when heated as in food processing, into ethylene thiourea which is classified as a 'probable human carcinogen' by the US Environmental Protection Agency.

Pesticide Poisoning

One of the most detailed analyses of the extent of acute pesticide poisoning has been carried out by the Regional Poisoning Treatment Centre at the Royal Infirmary in Edinburgh[109]. All admissions following acute exposures to pesticides over a 6-year period (1981–86) were identified. In the 6 years under review there were over 9000 acute poisoning admissions to the Centre, fifty-seven of which followed alleged exposure to pesticides (0.6% of the total).

Forty of these were men and 14 were women, with the majority in the 20–40 years age group. Thirty-eight of the admissions (28 men and 10 women) were due to parasuicide (suicide attempts or self-harm), while 16 (12 men and four women) were due to accidents. Only ten of the accidents were work related (Figure 5.2).

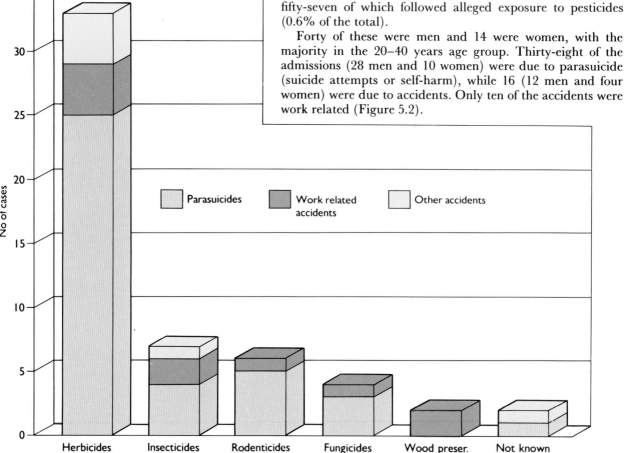

Figure 5.2
Cases of acute exposure to pesticides treated at the Edinburgh Royal Infirmary (1981–86).

Herbicides were involved in 33 of the 54 incidents (61%), and no fewer than 26 were due to paraquat (in parasuicide, not normal use). Ingestion was by far the most important route of exposure (46 cases) followed by inhalation (six cases) and the skin (two cases). In general, morbidity was either negligible or extreme. The majority of patients (41 out of 54) had no symptoms or relatively minor and short lived ones, such as nausea, vomiting, abdominal pain, diarrhoea, coughing and breathlessness. At the other extreme, the remaining 13 patients suffered life-threatening consequences, and ten of them died. None of the deaths and only one of the life-threatening illnesses resulted from work-related accidents.

There is a lack of information on the pattern and consequences of acute pesticide over-exposures in Britain. In 1985 the National Poisons Unit reported receiving 2270 enquiries[2]: These were, however, enquiries and not necessarily cases of actual poisoning or even exposure. Given these reservations, the Edinburgh study provides an invaluable snapshot of the low level of poisoning by pesticides in normal use in one part of the country. The data presented confirmed that acute incidents involving pesticides are an uncommon cause of admission to hospital. The number of admissions for pesticide poisoning as a percentage of the total number of admissions for possible poisoning is in keeping with the statistics for pesticide poisonings in England and Wales[110]. It might be argued that incidents would be unlikely to come to a city centre unit, but the catchment area of the Royal Infirmary includes areas where pesticides are extensively used, the agricultural lands of East Lothian and the Tweed valley.

The most obvious finding was that parasuicide is a much more common reason for adult pesticide admissions than accidents. Unfortunately, little can be done to prevent people deliberately harming themselves with pesticides if they really want to do so. It is, however, a cause for concern that none of those who killed themselves with paraquat should have had access to the formulation, which should only be sold to those engaged in the trade or business of agriculture, horticulture or forestry. It is illegal to supply concentrated paraquat except to farmers and so on, and the 20% solution is never available to the general public. The 20% formulation, Gramoxone, contains a dye to give a colour not associated with any drink, an emetic to cause vomiting if it is taken, and a potent stench. If people do drink it, it is a very deliberate act indeed.

The work-related accidents also give cause for concern, since

To prevent ingestion, Gramoxone, a 20% formulation of paraquat, contains unusually coloured dyes, induces vomiting and has a potent stench.

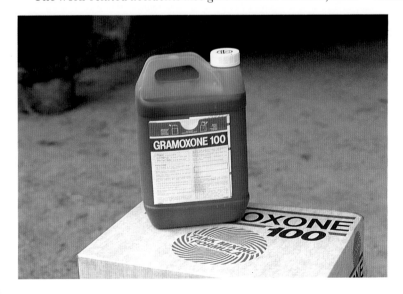

at least half of them were preventable with adequate training. Two were simply the result of stupidity (siphoning wood preservative, and removing the top of the bottle of paraquat with the teeth), and one a failure to apply common sense (eating a meal without washing after using a pesticide). However, a fourth resulted from a failure to comply with safety instructions supplied with the product, and a fifth from failure to maintain spray equipment in good working order.

The last two are as much a reflection of poor training, supervision and working practices as they are the fault of the workers themselves.

First Aid

It is clear from the Edinburgh study, as well as from national statistics, that admission for acute pesticide poisoning will not be a common occurrence in the accident and emergency department, still less for the general practitioner. Nevertheless, it is vital for the doctor or other person attending a person suspected of being a victim of pesticide poisoning to be able to take immediate steps to minimize the risk of serious injury. The Department of Health and Social Security has published a booklet on pesticide poisoning[111] which gives guidance to medical practitioners on the toxic effects of different classes of pesticides, and gives practical advice on treatment of acute poisoning. A new edition of the booklet is in preparation. The following first aid measures should be undertaken immediately in the case of pesticide poisoning:

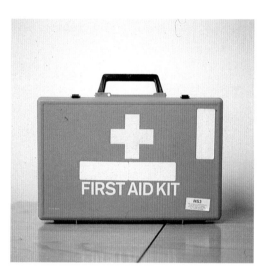

Administration of immediate and appropriate First Aid is vital for a victim of pesticide poisoning.

- Always remove the patient from the spraying area into shelter if possible.

- Keep the patient at rest.

- Remove all protective clothing and any other clothing that may be wet with the chemical, taking care not to contaminate yourself. Wash contaminated skin thoroughly with soap and cold water.

- If breathing ceases or weakens start artificial respiration immediately, making sure the airway is clear.

- If contaminated with pesticides, the eye should be copiously irrigated with clean water for at least 15 minutes with the eyelid held open and then be covered with a soft pad of sterilized cotton wool kept firmly in position by a shade or bandage.

- When the patient is being transported to hospital it is important to ensure that breathing is maintained, the airway kept clear and the inhalation of vomit prevented.

- Inform the hospital of the name of the chemical or preparation the patient has been using. Make available the label and other information on the container, as well as any product leaflets.

LONG-TERM HEALTH EFFECTS

Given today's extensive use of pesticides, both for agricultural and non-agricultural purposes, it is almost impossible for any member of the population to avoid daily exposure to very low levels of several different pesticides in food and water. Consequently there is concern about possible adverse effects on human health arising from continual long-term low-level exposure, that is the potential for chronic toxicity.

Chronic effects are only likely to become apparent after prolonged exposure to a chemical. In the case of cancer this may be a period of several decades which leads to difficulties in identifying the causative agent. The slower the onset of the effect, the more difficult it is to prove the particular cause for several reasons. Firstly, any individual will be exposed to a wide range of possible causative factors. Secondly, the extent and form of exposure to a particular suspect pesticide is unlikely to be known with any degree of accuracy. Thirdly, any effect has to show up against a background of 'natural' disease which is part of the process of ageing. Pesticides that produce a 'unique' disease in man are most likely to be identified, particularly if they produce a similar effect in animal species. Conversely, if a pesticide increased the incidence of a very common human disease, it might be almost impossible to identify the cause[2].

One way of attempting to identify the long-term, or chronic, effect of pesticides on health is by studying the different groups of people who are exposed to these chemicals in varying ways. The evidence relating to exposure in manufacturers, users and their families is particularly important in studying the effects of pesticides on the health of the individual.

The Pyramid of Exposure

Several groups in the population are subject to pesticide exposure. The hazards of pesticides affect workers, workers' families, and the general public, in order of decreasing exposure but greatly increasing population at risk. These risks have been expressed as a pyramid of exposure (Figure 5.3).

The people at the apex of the pyramid, relatively small in number but subject to a high risk of exposure, are workers in the pesticide industry: manufacturers, formulators, packers, and distributors. In 1987 the Chairman of the House of Commons Select Committee on Pesticides[2] considered that under-reporting of pesticide incidents through organizational, resource and medical diagnosis problems was a major obstacle in the full assessment of pesticide health hazards.

The most accurate data concerning pesticide poisoning come from California, where the state covers farm workers under its Workers' Compensation law and requires physicians to report pesticide poisoning when applying for reimbursement. Figures for the 1970s suggest that risks have declined for applicators, probably due to improved awareness and safer practices.

Risks to Manufacturers

A comprehensive overview of delayed health hazards of pesticide exposure is given in the review by Sharp and

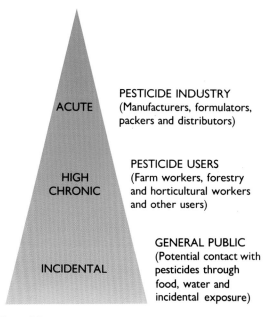

Figure 5.3
Pyramid of exposure.

colleagues, published in the *Annual Review of Public Health* in 1986[112]. One hundred and seventy-eight studies were reviewed. Epidemiological evidence provides the focus, but in some cases pertinent animal and clinical research is presented to support or contrast with epidemiological conclusions. The authors identified several lines of enquiry: farming occupations, pest control operators and other workers (including manufacturers) with a known exposure to pesticides. Specific agents of concern for cancer are phenoxy herbicides and related compounds, dioxin impurities, arsenicals and organochlorines such as DDT.

Several US studies reviewed by Sharp *et al* have examined the long-term health status of workers in pesticide manufacturing facilities. Three studies of workers potentially exposed to phenoxy herbicides and their contaminant (the dioxin 2,3,7,8-TCDD) revealed that although exposure was high (signified by the development of chloracne in most workers, a symptom associated with high exposure to TCDD), no adverse mortality rates were detected[113–115]. Although the cohort size of the industrial populations were small and the follow-up period in one of the studies may have been insufficient to detect an adverse effect, all three studies failed to reveal any significantly increased cancer rates in the populations studied. A more detailed study of over 5,000 workers in a UK facility manufacturing phenoxy herbicides also failed to reveal any adverse health effects[116]. Another recent study of over 3000 Danish phenoxy herbicide manufacturers largely supported the lack of health effects, apart from an increased incidence of soft tissue sarcomas which could neither be linked to degree nor duration of exposure[117]. One study commented on an increased prevalence of premalignant skin lesions amongst 4,4'-bipyridyl (an intermediate compound used in the manufacture of paraquat) manufacturing workers in Taiwan[118] but suggested that sunlight was a necessary cofactor.

Other mortality studies of the manufacturers of chlorinated hydrocarbon pesticides (chlordane, heptachlor, endrin, aldrin, dieldrin, DDT) and captan do not show any increased cancer risk for any particular site or an overall cancer risk. An increased risk of lung cancer does appear to be associated with manufacturers of inorganic arsenicals. Studies on the manufacturers of EDB and 4,4'-bipyridyl are inconclusive as to the compounds' carcinogenic potential.

Studies on the morbidity experience of manufacturers of pesticides have shown that chlorinated hydrocarbon pesticides appear to be without long-term effect. Organophosphate pesticides may alter haematological profiles and blood biochemistry normal values, but to what morbidological significance remains open to speculation. Manufacture of 4,4'-bipyridyl appears to be positively associated with premalignant skin lesions and, therefore, must be a cause for concern. The absence of any long-term neurotoxicological effect from several chemicals, including chlordecone, chlorpyrifos and pentachlorophenol is reassuring, while the effects of 2,4-D and 2,4,5-T remain unconfirmed. The only agricultural product that appears to have a permanent adverse effect on reproductive processes is DBCP[68]. High chlordecone exposure may have a transitory effect on sperm production. The overall morbidity among manufacturers of pesticides appears to be closely similar to that in other manufacturing industries, and it is reassuring that various pesticides do not appear to represent classes of chemicals that are unduly hazardous in other industries.

Nevertheless, while the results of the epidemiological surveys available are reassuring, no studies have been carried out on the workers engaged in the manufacture of many pesticides. 'Absence of evidence is not evidence of absence'[83]. Further evidence is required and employers, trade unions and individual workers need to maintain their vigilance with regard to health and safety procedures.

Risks to Users

In 1986 three UK trade unions (TGWU, GMB and NUPE) carried out a survey of unionized pesticide operators[119]. These included farm-workers, local authority grounds staff, parks and gardens staff, nursery workers, and Forestry Commission staff. It is likely that those who responded would be those who felt they had a problem (known as 'motivational bias' in epidemiology); but in the absence of any similar UK survey, the results should be taken as indicative of work practices and health problems experienced by pesticide users in the UK. Fifty per cent of respondents reported that they had suffered symptoms (headaches, sickness, sore throats) that they attributed to exposure to pesticides. This was despite the fact that a large proportion (greater than 80%) were being supplied with and wore protective equipment and clothing. Thirty-eight per cent of the respondents had received no training on the health and safety aspects of the use of pesticides, and 50% said that their safety representatives had received no information from their employers on pesticide hazards.

It is worth noting that this survey concentrated on unionized workers. A survey including pesticide users who are not trade union members, for example agricultural workers on small farms, would probably have uncovered a more rudimentary adherence to good health and safety practice[120]. IIt is true also that the symptoms reported could have been caused by other factors (for example, headaches from driving a tractor on a hot day, sore throats from applying pesticides in the hay fever season, or nausea from the smell of some pesticides). The survey was carried out before the Food and Environment Protection Act (FEPA) was passed in 1985, which makes statutory the wording on pesticide labels. The label contains all the necessary information about protective clothing, and it is illegal for a farm-worker to use a pesticide without this specified protection. The FEPA provisions are now supplemented by the COSHH regulations.

Three major areas have been subjects of study into the possible effects of long-term pesticide exposure: cancer; reproductive hazards; and neurological disorders.

Cancer

Many studies seeking to identify possible links between cancer and pesticides have been published. The specific agents of primary concern have been phenoxy herbicides and related compounds, dioxin impurities, arsenicals, and organochlorines such as DDT; and these have been the focus of case studies and

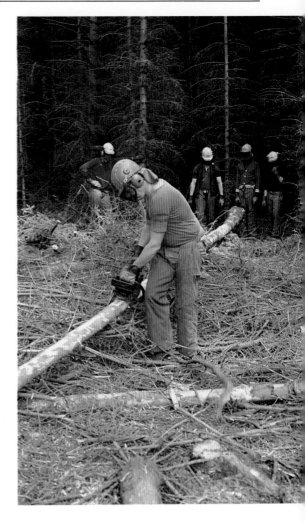

A health and safety study of Forestry Commission staff, and other operators, revealed that more than a third had not received health and safety training on the use of pesticides.

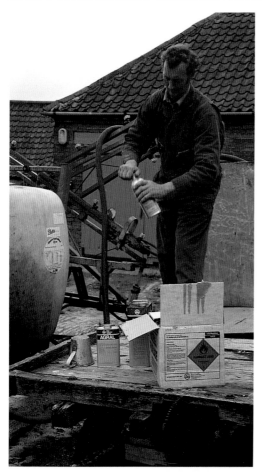

It is a legal requirement for users of pesticides to wear protective clothing as recommended on the label. This farm worker should be wearing coverall, gloves and face shield.

epidemiological investigations in the USA, New Zealand, UK and Sweden. The most consistent line of enquiry into the carcinogenicity of pesticides has been the studies of farming occupations. These have been well summarized in probably the most extensive review of chronic health effects of pesticides by Sharp and colleagues in 1986[112] and are reproduced in Table 5.1.

In the USA interest in the long-term health effects of pesticide exposure, particularly carcinogenicity, has focused strongly on agricultural workers. Such attention is appropriate because this largely independent group of workers has virtually no protection under the US Occupational Health and Safety Administration and has, particularly since the 1960s, had potentially large exposures to pesticides. In 1988 the Council on Scientific Affairs of the American Medical Association (AMA) published a review of the available literature on the potential carcinogenicity of pesticides[121] and called on the AMA, through its scientific journals and publications, to alert physicians to the potential hazards of agricultural pesticides, and to provide physicians with advice on such hazards for their patients.

As the AMA report recognizes, the potential effects of widespread, chronic low-level exposure to pesticides is only partially understood. At one time farmers were thought to have a lower overall mortality than other workers because they were presumed to have a healthy lifestyle. Numerous studies[122–124] now suggest that today's farmers and farm workers could have an increased risk of developing certain types of cancers, and the question is whether pesticides play a role. Some investigators have reported that agricultural workers have higher death rates from malignant brain tumours[125]; agricultural workers and pesticide applicators have also been shown to have increased risk for testicular cancer[126].

The 'farmer studies' have generally shown an increased level of certain cancers in agricultural occupations. The studies listed above demonstrated elevated relative risks for farmers and similar workers, particularly of leukaemia, myeloma, Hodgkin's and non-Hodgkin's lymphomas. This does not mean that contact with pesticides can be identified as the causative factor. In fact, several studies found significant associations between exposure to poultry and leukaemias and lymphomas[125,127–140]. There is certainly the possibility here of an interaction between agents, and there is some indirect evidence of leukaemias and lymphomas being mediated by viruses[110]. The whole issue of exposure to multiple agents, such as viruses and chemicals and their interaction requires further investigation.

Studies have been made of applicators of phenoxy herbicides. In 1977 Hardell[141] noted that five patients in a series of seven cases of mesenchymal tumours had had extensive exposure to phenoxy herbicides. This paper heralded a protracted exchange of correspondence in the *Lancet*[142] and reflected an emerging body of evidence from the 'Swedish Studies'. In 1974 Axelson and Sundell[143] examined a cohort of railway workers engaged in brush control. Between 1957 and 1972 six cases of cancer were detected in 207 workers exposed for at least 45 days to herbicides. While statistically significant increases in rates were noted in those workers exposed to amitrole, none was

Region	Outcome	Type of activity
California	Leukaemia,	Farming
	Hodgkin's lymphoma,	Farming
	multiple myeloma	Farming
Washington	Leukaemia,	Poultry
	multiple myeloma	Farming
South-east USA	Multiple myeloma,	Poultry
	uterine cervix,	Farming
	ovarian cancer	Farming
Nebraska	Leukaemia	Corn, insecticide, poultry, cattle, hogs
Texas	Leukaemia	Farming
Iowa	Leukaemia,	Farming
	lymphoma,	Farming
	multiple myeloma,	Farming
	prostatic cancer,	Farming
	stomach cancer	Farming
Iowa	Leukaemia	Poultry, herbicides
Wisconsin	Lymphosarcoma,	None noted
	reticulum cell sarcoma	Cattle dairy, small grains, insecticides, wheat
Iowa	Multiple myeloma,	Poultry, hogs, insecticides, herbicides
	non-Hodgkin's lymphoma,	Poultry, hogs, herbicides, milk production
	prostatic cancer,	None noted
	stomach cancer	Corn, cattle, milk production
Britain	Soft-tissue sarcoma	Farming
Illinois	non-Hodgkin's lymphoma,	Farming
	prostatic cancer	Farming
Wisconsin	Multiple myeloma	Poultry, insecticides, fertilizers
North Carolina	Melanoma,	Whites: poultry, cattle, dairying
		Whites: poultry, cattle
	prostatic cancer,	Non-whites: peanuts, chemical use
	brain cancer,	Non-whites: corn, tobacco, peanuts, chemicals
	non-Hodgkin's lymphoma, leukaemia	Non-whites: none noted
New Zealand	Lymphoma,	Farming
	multiple myeloma,	Farming
	both	Orchard (poultry)

Table 5.1
Summary of studies investigating possible links between cancer and pesticide use among farmers

Source: Sharp D. S. et al. Delayed health hazards of pesticide exposure. Annual Review of Public Health 1986; 7:41–71

noted for those exposed to any of the phenoxy herbicides. In 1980 Axelson et al.[144] updated the cohort and noted an excess of tumours in workers exposed to both amitrole and phenoxy herbicides. The earlier indication that amitrole alone was the factor associated with an increased incidence of cancer was not confirmed in the updated study.

In 1979 Hardell and Sandstrom[145] published results of a case control study of 52 cases of soft-tissue sarcoma, registered from three northern countries in Sweden. A detailed assessment of exposure to specific phenoxy herbicides such as 2,4,5-T, 2,4-D and MCPA was undertaken by questionnaire. People with soft-tissue carcinoma were 5.7 times more likely to have been exposed than those who were not, but in most cases exposure was to multiple agents[145]. In a 1982 article[146] Hay has argued that because 2,4-D is often contaminated with dioxins, it may well be the contaminant which is the cause for concern. Hardell *et al.*[147] then extended their studies to include malignant lymphomas, demonstrating in 169 cases with 388 controls, that the ratio of exposed to controls was 5.3. When exposure to only phenoxy herbicides was examined, the ratio remained at a significant 4.8. These studies thus suggested that exposed workers ran 5–6 times the risk of developing lymphomas and soft-tissue sarcomas.

In 1986, a major National Cancer Institute study[148,149] into farm workers in Kansas supported the findings of the Swedish investigations for non-Hodgkin's lymphoma, but not soft-tissue sarcomas or Hodgkin's disease. The relative risk of developing non-Hodgkin's lymphoma (NHL) increased significantly in association with the number of days per year exposed to herbicides and to the latent period. Men exposed to herbicides more than 20 days per year had a sixfold increase of NHL. Frequent users who mixed or applied the herbicides themselves, were at eight times the risk relative to non-farmers. The increased risk was particularly associated with use of phenoxyacetic acid herbicides, specifically 2,4-D.

Neither phenoxy herbicides nor their potential contaminants (dioxins) can be unequivocally stated to cause cancer in humans. The studies undertaken in Sweden in the 1970s[142–144], as outlined above, provide the strongest evidence of causality in humans. Three other case control studies, similar in size and methodology were conducted in New Zealand and found non-increased risk for all three cancer sites with exposure to phenoxy herbicides[136]. Inconsistent findings such as these are unlikely if there is a true causal relationship, and the possibility has been raised that different levels of dioxin contamination of phenoxy herbicides in the two countries may be a factor. Swedish populations may be exposed to two necessary agents (one being phenoxy herbicides or dioxin contaminants) that cause cancer; those in New Zealand may not be exposed to the second factor. Another possibility relates to the pattern of spraying. Because of the climate, spraying in Sweden is carried out intensively over a 2–3 month period, whereas spraying in New Zealand (as in the UK and USA) occurs intermittently over a longer period. This may mean that Swedish workers receive a relatively high absorbed dose in a shorter period of time.

Although the connection with pesticides seems strongest with lymphomas, myeloma, leukaemia, and soft tissue sarcomas, there is also evidence of a relationship with other types of cancer. Significantly higher rates of lung cancer were recorded in a cohort of 1658 agricultural workers using pesticides in Germany between 1948 and 1972[140]. The increased risk was independent of whether or not workers smoked. The longer employees had worked with pesticides, the more likely they were to develop lung cancer. Similar findings for lung cancer were recorded in a 1983 study of pesticide applicators in Florida[150]. This time it was not possible to assess the smoking habits of the workers.

The carcinogenic potential of arsenic, having been suspected for almost a century, is well established. Arsenical pesticides are rarely used nowadays for this reason, but a link between exposure in the past to arsenical pesticides and the development of respiratory cancers has been demonstrated[151].

There is less evidence of a causal relationship between pesticides and cancers of the digestive and urinary systems. Hardell examined rates for colon cancer as part of a series of studies in Sweden and although there was a very slight increase in risk for those exposed to herbicides in their work, this was not statistically significant[152]. However, Thiess and colleagues[153] did find an excess of stomach cancer in a group of 74 workers accidentally exposed to dioxins. A study of Vietnam veterans in Massachusetts[154] demonstrated significantly greater numbers of cases of kidney cancer on the death certificates of personnel exposed to Agent Orange, but as with all the Vietnam studies a longer period of follow-up is needed. The link between bladder cancer and the use in the 1940s and 1950s of the rodenticide ANTU (or a contaminant found in it) now seems strong, and ANTU was withdrawn from use in the UK in 1967.

Despite the accumulation of evidence in specific areas, the conclusion that has to be reached is that the epidemiological evidence has so far been insufficient to demonstrate clear causal relationships between most pesticides and cancer[155,156].

Reproduction

Studies of the effects of pesticides on fertility and fetal development are in principle much simpler to conduct than investigations into cancer, because the at-risk population is more readily identified, and the period both of exposure and for identification of any adverse effect is much shorter[2]. This is an area where public concern may be even greater than it is about possible carcinogenic effects. As with the perceived risk of smoking, the possibility of developing cancer 20 years after exposure to pesticides may be taken less seriously than the possibility of giving birth to a handicapped child in the much shorter term. Nonetheless, there has been a paucity of studies into the effects of pesticide exposure on human reproduction. Only a few chemicals have been associated positively with birth defects in man, for example mercury, lead and thalidomide; much of the concern that has been expressed about pesticides stems from animal findings into the teratogenic properties of chemicals. In a review of the literature, the London Food Commission has listed 35 pesticides that have been linked with possible reproductive effects in animals. The pesticides include widely used formulations, such as aldrin, benomyl, captan, carbaryl, dieldrin, dinoseb, ioxynil, lindane, maneb, and paraquat. The sources for most of these data are *Dangerous Properties of Industrial Materials*[157] and the Equal Opportunities Commission's *Reproductive Hazards at Work*[158].

Dibromochloroproprane (DBCP) is the pesticide most clearly implicated in the impairment of fertility. Interest in the reproductive effects of DBCP was sparked when wives of workers in a northern California manufacturing plant complained of an inability to become pregnant. Studies by Whorton and colleagues[68] showed that almost half the workers had lower than normal sperm counts, compared with less than 10% in non-exposed workers. Subsequent studies have confirmed that the degree and length of exposure to DBCP is directly related to reduced sperm count. It has also been suggested that there is a preponderance of female offspring in men exposed to DBCP; there have been no studies of the offspring of women who have been exposed to the chemical.

Not surprisingly there has been enormous public concern in the USA about the exposure of US servicemen to Agent Orange (2,4,5-T contaminated with dioxin), used as a defoliant in Vietnam, and its possible effects on their offspring[159]. Nevertheless, studies of veterans in the USA, Australia and Vietnam have been largely inconclusive. The US Air Force is currently following a cohort of over 1000 men (The Ranch Hands) who flew aircraft that sprayed Agent Orange. The initial findings[160] showed no differences between the Ranch Hands and unexposed veterans in semen quality and number of children fathered. However, the study has found a significant increase in miscarriage rate, a higher overall rate of birth defects and a larger number of neonatal deaths in the period following exposure compared with the period before. A review of unpublished studies by Hatch[161] also claimed an increased risk for birth defects, particularly of the neural tube and facial clefts, in the children of fathers who served in South Vietnam. Another of the studies reviewed wives of servicemen who had twice the number of miscarriages than might have been expected (16% of pregnancies compared with 8.5%).

The US Centers for Disease Control were mandated by the US Congress to carry out an extensive review of the health status of Vietnam veterans. The Vietnam Experience Study involved interviewing 7924 Vietnam and 7364 non-Vietnam veterans who had entered the US army from 1965 to 1971. During telephone interviews the Vietnam veterans reported many more adverse reproductive and child health outcomes than did the non-Vietnam veterans. However, examination of hospital records told a different story. The children of the Vietnam veterans were no more likely to have birth defects recorded on hospital birth records[162]. A study carried out at the Boston Hospital for Women also suggested that the risk of spontaneous abortion was not increased in women married to Vietnam veterans[163].

Despite the extensive studies into the families of men exposed to Agent Orange, the results of a paternally mediated adverse effect on reproductive outcome has not been established. It is even more difficult to establish a maternally mediated effect due to the numerous factors that can influence reproductive outcome, for example maternal age, smoking habits, and heavy work during pregnancy.

Studies of the effects of Agent Orange exposure on the unfortunate people of Vietnam have been far fewer, hampered as they are by inaccurate records both of exposure and birth details. Two studies[164,165] have found significant increases in congenital malformations of the neural tube and the palate in the children of Vietnamese civilians. Peaks in the relative frequency of spina bifida and cleft palate coincided with the 2 years of particularly heavy spraying (1967 and 1968). There were also almost twice the rate of molar pregnancies (hydatidiform mole) in the heavy spraying years, and the highest rate of stillbirths (68 per 1000) was in the province of Tay Ninh, an area heavily exposed.

Although DDT is no longer used in most parts of the world, its residues are persistent. Organochlorine pesticides such as DDT pass through the placenta, with an average level in the newborn blood reaching around a third of that in maternal blood. Limited evidence suggests that DDT is related to miscarriage and premature delivery. It has been suggested that organochlorine pesticides have weak oestrogenic effects and may precipitate labour. The problem is most evident in the Third World where exposure to DDT continues. Studies in Brazil[166] and India[167] have shown DDT levels significantly higher in the cord blood of preterm infants than in term infants. In the Indian case, the levels were five times higher and the highest levels were seen in the most premature infants.

Neurological Disorders

The nervous system has been recognized as a target organ for pesticide toxicity for several decades. Indeed, the desired pesticidal action of the organophosphates is based on the same principle as 'nerve gases' used in chemical warfare. In addition to the neurological signs and symptoms of acute intoxication, organophosphates may cause two delayed effects from acute high dose or chronic low dose exposure: delayed polyneuropathy, and neurobehavioural effects. Three cases of permanent polyneuropathy due to organophosphorus pesticide poisoning were recorded in the UK in 1952. Follow-up studies of the survivors of acute pesticide poisoning episodes suggest that a few people may continue to experience persistent neurobehavioural symptoms. A group of 117 workers examined 3 years after systemic poisoning by organophosphates were found to have continued visual disturbances, gastrointestinal symptoms, headaches and nervousness[168]. Possible long-term neurological effects have also been associated with short-term exposure to the grain fumigant methyl bromide[2].

The effects of pesticides on the nervous system can be difficult to detect[169]. In one epidemiological study of matched pairs of previously acutely organophosphate-poisoned individuals and non-poisoned controls it was concluded that, whereas there was little difference found in the more obvious clinical tests, there were many differences found in more subtle, neuropsychological tests.

Risks to Workers' Families

The families of farm workers are exposed to pesticide residues on equipment, garments, containers and in their homes. Children are exposed by playing or working in the fields; they may be particularly at risk because of their body size and their eating and dressing habits[170]. Children work on farms everywhere in the world and are at high risk of accidents[120]. Pesticide hazards for farm-workers, their families and children are particularly great in the Third World, where hundreds of millions of peasants not only work but live in the fields from infancy to old age. In the USA, Congress banned child labour (under 12 years of age) in 1974, but 3 years later relented and allowed the US Department of Labour (DOL) to make exceptions for some agricultural work, including helping at harvest time[171].

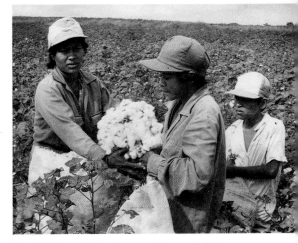

Pesticide hazards for farm-workers and their families are particularly great in the Third World, where peasants not only work, but live in the fields, from infancy to old age.

Environmental Protection Agency regulations and the supervision provided by farmers and growers were deemed insufficient to protect children from pesticide hazards. Therefore DOL issued a list of chemicals and procedures expected to be safe for children. The list was amended twice between 1978 and 1979 under pressure from growers who wished to spray unlisted chemicals and to employ children. The DOL regulations were challenged by the National Association of Farmworkers Organisation and were invalidated in 1980 by the US Court of Appeal as incompatible with DOL's duty under the Fair Labour Standards Act. The US Department of Agriculture estimates that 800000 children under the age of 16 still work in the fields[171,172].

Agricultural workers' wives could be exposed to higher levels of pesticides than women in other parts of the community. Exposure could possibly occur in the home from washing contaminated clothing, and when women are working alongside men in the fields. Women are subject not only to similar risks of cancer and other health effects as men, but there is also the problem of teratogenicity, the effect on the unborn child. Women who either live in a high agricultural activity area, or who work with pesticides, appear to show conflicting results for a possible association with pesticide exposure and malformed offspring. The results from the studies into the teratogenic effects of pesticides have been limited by small numbers and by recall of pregnancies up to 30 years previously. A bias in recall may also operate, in that a woman bearing a healthy child may not remember if, or to what, she was exposed, since her pregnancy was normal. As was observed at a WHO meeting on the effects of occupational factors on reproduction[173], a relatively large number of papers have been published on reproductive function, following exposure to chemicals in the work environment. In most of the papers the methods used were scientifically so poor that relatively few definite conclusions can be reached. However, a study by Schwartz and Logerfo[174] in California found that there was no increased risk of limb malformations for parental involvement in agricultural work; although maternal residence in a country of high agricultural activity and pesticide use was associated with an increased risk. This study indicated that exposure to pesticides and other agents associated with high agricultural activity in the residential environment, but not in the working environment, may be associated with an increased risk of congenital limb defects. Conversely, a more recent study in Canada by MacDonald *et al.*[175] found that occupation in pesticide/horticulture was associated with an increased risk of congenital malformations, but that exposure to pesticides *per se* was not associated with an increased risk. Other studies have reported an increased risk of cleft lip and palate in rural agriculturally intensive areas in the USA[176], while in Australia a significant association of congenital limb defects was reported with exposure of women to pesticides both in the residential and occupational environment. A greater risk was associated with exposures where women were in close proximity, usually in a work setting[177].

The reproductive outcomes of couples with paternal exposure to agrochemicals has also been extensively researched. A study in 1983[178] compared rates of spina bifida, anencephaly and facial clefts for offspring of fathers whose job title suggested exposure to agricultural chemicals (for example, farmers, and gardeners) with rates in children of fathers in other occupations. Defect rates were considerably higher for a variety of agricultural occupations. However, a case control study by Golding and Sladden[179] published the same year failed to confirm these findings.

Particularly in the light of the Seveso accident, there has been interest in whether women who have worked, or whose husbands have worked with chlorophenols have a higher rate of infants with congenital malformations, miscarriages, stillbirths or infant deaths. This does not seem to be the case. Smith and colleagues[180] compared reproductive histories of pesticide applicators (mostly 2,4,5-T) in New Zealand with those of agricultural contractors. Wives often also worked with their husbands in the fields. The researchers found no difference in congenital malformations, stillbirths, miscarriages and overall fertility rates. Even where men had significant levels of exposure to a contaminant, TCDD, as evidenced by chloracne, there has been little evidence of an increase in fathering infants with congenital abnormalities[181,182].

Vietnam war veterans exposed to Agent Orange (a mixture of the two herbicides, 2,4-D and 2,4,5-T, containing up to 30 parts per million TCDD) have been studied extensively for deleterious reproductive performance and outcomes. A review of three large epidemiology studies[183] – one by the Australian Government, one by the Atlanta Centre for Birth Defects and one by the US Air Force – on men who had carried out defoliation missions in Vietnam, concluded that service in Vietnam and, therefore, possible exposure to Agent Orange did not of itself raise the risk of fathering a malformed offspring.

In conclusion, there is no evidence to support a paternally mediated effect on offspring following exposure to the phenoxyherbicides.

Summary of Studies of Pesticide Users

Studies on the mortality experience of pesticide applicators have shown that chronic poisoning with lead arsenate may be associated with lung tumours and skin lesions[184]. However, several studies did not find an association between exposure and increased lung tumour incidences[185–187], so that it is postulated that poisoning – thereby initiating a primary toxic response – is a prerequisite for subsequent development of lung tumours. The soil fumigant 1,3-dichloropropene has been associated with several case reports of leukaemia[188] while exposure to triazines[189], chlordane[190], heptachlor[191] and other organochlorine[192] pesticides do not appear to be carcinogenic in man.

Exposure to phenoxy herbicides (2,4-D, 2,4,5-T, MCPA and contaminants) and chlorophenols constitute the majority of studies of defined exposure to either applicators or farmers. Results from studies are inconclusive with respect to an association with Hodgkin's disease[193–199], leukaemia and soft-tissue sarcomas[116,193–197,200–202]. However, there does appear to be an association between exposure to these compounds and non-Hodgkin's lymphoma[196,197].

Other studies, where exposure data were lacking, revealed that farmers were at an increased risk from cancers of the stomach, prostate, leukaemia, multiple myeloma, and non-Hodgkin's lymphoma, but at a decreased risk from cancers of the liver, lung, colon, oesophagus, larynx, pancreas and kidney. No excessive risk was associated with agricultural workers/applicators and testicular cancer. Brain gliomas were tentatively linked to fungicide and insecticide use[127-129,203-215].

The morbidity studies of personnel exposed to agrochemicals by application and use of the products show that high blood organochlorine levels may be associated with the development of hypertension and arteriosclerosis, but do not affect other chronic disease conditions[192]. Haematological profiles can be altered by high exposure to organochlorine[216] and organophosphate compounds, but not following exposure to deltamethrin[217] or paraquat[218]. The relevance of this observation is unknown. Other morbidity studies have shown equivocal and inconsistent associations between exposure to chlordane[219], heptachlor[219] and DDT[220] with blood dyscrasias including leukaemia.

Organophosphates depress cholinesterase activity in a dose-dependent relationship[221-223], but do not appear to cause chronic neurotoxicity[224]. EDB does not cause chromosomal damage[225], but organochlorine and organophosphate pesticides in specific combinations do appear to cause an increased number of chromatid breaks[226].

Past exposure levels, and currently monitored urinalysis, do not appear to be causing an increased risk for cancer from chlordimeform exposure[227].

Skin effects are an occupational hazard for agricultural workers[228] and many specific compounds have been implicated, for example, anilazine[229], fenvalerate[230], and deltamethrin[217]. With respect to the respiratory system, 'farmer's lung' (hypersensitivity pneumonitis) is also an occupational hazard, but is not related to agrochemical exposure[231,232]. Paraquat has no effect on respiratory health[218]. Fruit growers exposed to an average of 13 different compounds during a single spraying season appear to have suffered an adverse respiratory health effect, but the causative agents are unknown[233].

Effects on reproduction do not appear to be an occupational hazard for agricultural male workers[234-237], but organochlorine and organophosphates in specific combinations did appear to increase the miscarriage rate, stillbirth rate and infertility in a selected population where both partners were exposed to the pesticides[226]. 2,4,5-T is free from implication of adverse reproductive health in males[235,236]. Maternal occupation in agriculture, but not exposure to pesticides, has been implicated in a risk for congenital developmental effects[238].

In conclusion, skin diseases appear to be the main cause of adverse health effects in applicators of agrochemicals. Hypersensitivity pneumonitis does appear to be an occupational hazard for farmers, but this is not related to pesticide exposure. No adverse respiratory effects or reproductive effects can be related to specific exposures to specific pesticides. The morbidity experience of pesticide applicators does not appear to be outstanding or markedly different from any other occupation that involves exposure to a variety of different chemical products.

The 1987 Agriculture Committee[2] considered the acute and chronic health effects of exposure to pesticides in great detail, taking evidence from a wide variety of interested bodies. The report published by the Committee Chairman forms a useful summary of the problem. On acute poisoning hazards the Committee were made well aware that such incidents do occur, however rarely. But the systems for collecting data relating to exposure incidents were felt to be woefully inadequate. Further, there should be prompt and effective follow-up investigations of all reports of serious exposure.

On the chronic effects, it was recognized that most studies have been inconclusive. However, public anxiety can no longer be allayed by merely stating that no harmful effects have been observed from a particular pesticide and therefore it is safe. Those responsible for the clearance of pesticides must convince the public that they have the resources, knowledge and independence of judgement to investigate potential risk to human health from pesticide use – and they must do this more openly.

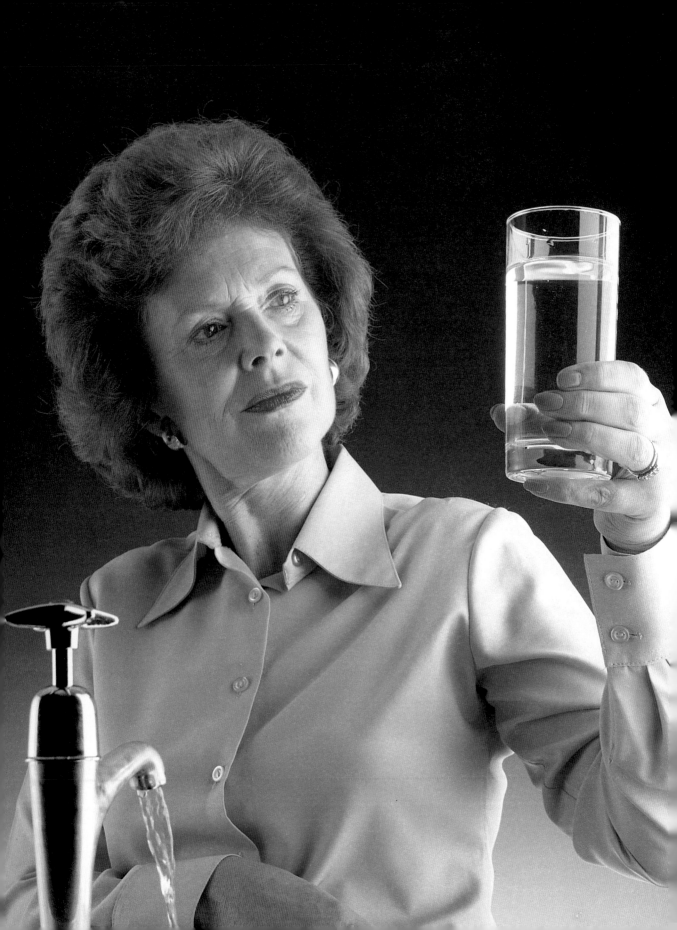

6 EFFECTS ON HEALTH IN THE COMMUNITY

Pesticides have undoubtedly brought us benefits in food production and public health. But with those benefits have come risks; risks to manufacturers, users, consumers, and the wider public. No chemical can ever be totally safe, let alone those that are designed to be toxic to some forms of life. From government to amateur gardener, we weigh up these risks and benefits in deciding whether or not a pesticide is to be used, using the information that is available to us.

THE IDEA OF RISK

We all have a general idea of what 'risk' means. We are familiar with the idea from childhood. We risk burning our hands if we touch the stove. We risk skinning our knees if we ride our bikes too fast. So we learn to modify our behaviour, taking into account the risks as we work out the best ways to enjoy ourselves[239]. In adult life we weigh up risks and benefits when taking many of the decisions of everyday life. Should we have our child vaccinated? Should I change career? Should we buy that house near the nuclear power station? Should I drive home after another drink?

The word risk is probably derived from the Greek word 'rhiza', the hazards of sailing too near to the cliffs. The idea of risk and its management was well understood by the ancient Greeks and Romans, who identified many common hazards and potentially effective ways of minimizing their capacity to cause harm. The Roman writer Vitruvius observed, well before the birth of Christ, that workers exposed to the fumes of molten lead suffered disorders of the blood and concluded that water should not be carried in lead pipes if it was to be wholesome[240]. However, following the decline of the Greek and Roman civilizations, there was little progress for centuries towards the greater understanding of the links between hazards and harm. Few could comprehend basic biological and physical processes. Techniques for the systematic collection and analysis of data were yet to emerge. The scientific principles of formal experimentation were hardly developed at all. As we have seen in the first chapter, the medieval world picture was one of arbitrary events, endured with fatalism. It was not until Blaise Pascal laid the foundations for the theory of probability in the mid-seventeenth century that a true revolution in intellectual development became possible. The likelihood that events would come to pass became a subject for scientists, not soothsayers[241].

The concept of probability brought logic to the study of the likelihood of events, frequencies and averages. In the practical

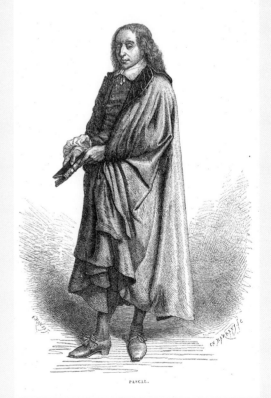

Blaise Pascal.

competitive world of commerce an emerging class of merchants needed to be able to calculate more precisely whether a planned venture would make or lose money: its risk, in other words. Mathematical theories of probability were soon being employed to show how long people might be expected to live, and so the practice of life assurance received its foundations. These developments created a far better understanding of the incidence and distribution of disease and injury in the community. There were increasing numbers of studies aimed at identifying cause-and-effect relationships between the things people do and the adverse health effects that could result. By the end of the nineteenth century the following linkages had been demonstrated[239]:

1 London smog and respiratory disease.
2 Tobacco snuff and cancer of the lining of the nose.
3 Child chimney sweeps and cancer of the scrotum.
4 Arsenic and cancer.
5 Aromatic amines and cancer of the bladder.
6 Sunlight and skin cancer.
7 Contaminated water and cholera.
8 Slum living and general ill health.

Risk Assessment and Risk Management

Although the concept of risk is familiar to us all, the term is also used in a more technical way by scientists. The way in which most scientists believe the word should be used[242] is as an expression of probability – the likelihood that something unpleasant will happen. More precisely, risk can be defined as the measured or estimated probability of injury, disease or death inherent in our daily activities[243]. A hazard is a set of circumstances that may cause harmful consequences, and the likelihood of its doing so is the risk associated with it. There are many kinds of losses resulting from many kinds of hazards. Losses can be represented as costs to society, and costs are also incurred when we try to reduce risks. But the degree of risk can be managed. The probability that occurrences may cause harm can be increased or decreased by the influence of risk factors.

Estimation of the risk associated with the use of chemicals requires identification of the potential health effects (toxicity) as well as the amount and possible ways through which a person might come into contact with the substance (exposure). One difficulty is that for many chemicals we do not know exactly what that toxicity is likely to be. It is the combination of both toxicity and exposure that must be considered for determination of risk. We might say:

$$\text{Risk} = \text{Hazard} \times \text{Exposure}$$

If we really want to understand how important a risk is, we need to express it in quantitative terms. This is where the science of risk assessment comes in. Risk assessment may be defined as the process of determining the probability that exposure to a compound will have an adverse effect on a given biological system[244]. The process of risk assessment depends for its success on the availability of plentiful and accurate data, and is often divided into:

1 *Risk estimation* (quantitative estimates) which relies on scientific activity and judgement. Statistically significant numbers of previous incidents can be used to predict both the magnitude and the likelihood (the risk) of harmful events in the future.
2 *Risk evaluation* (qualitative estimates) which relies on social and political judgements to determine the importance of hazards and the risk of harm, from the point of view of the individual and the community. This aspect of risk assessment includes the perception of risk, and the trading-off of perceived risks and benefits[239].

As it is not possible to eliminate all involuntary risk in our lives, governments, administrative bodies and the managers of large industrial installations must be able to identify significant risks to society, and then to establish appropriate control of those risks to acceptable levels. This process is called 'risk management'. Risk management takes place on an individual and a community level. For those actions considered voluntary, the individual can and does make deliberate choices in the lifestyle he or she adopts (for example, in decisions relating to smoking and alcohol, occupational health, transport and recreation). Access to information is central to the individual being able to make those choices. For those actions over which the individual has little control, society has come to expect government institutions to provide guidance in the form of regulatory actions.

Public Perception of Risk

In a democratic society several groups will be involved in decisions about risk. Some people belong to more than one group, but broadly they fall into one of three categories: the general public; their political representatives; and experts and managers. In principle, experts gather scientific evidence and give technical advice to politicians, who then legislate and regulate for the benefit and with the implicit agreement of the public. In practice things do not work out that way, and risk management in the manufacture and use of pesticides is as good an example as any. Risk management is not always as precise a procedure as politicians and the public would like: politicians have their own personal and partisan aims; the public may mistrust expert opinion; and for their part experts are inclined to dismiss the understanding of pressure groups and the wider public as insufficient for rational decision making[239].

The public are generally supposed to mistrust politicians and experts. In fact, a 1985 MORI Opinion Poll suggests they make quite fine distinctions about who is to be trusted on scientific and technological developments (Figure 6.1). Doctors are trusted sources of advice (67% trust, 10% not trust), members of Parliament at the other extreme, are treated with suspicion (11% trust, 63% not trust). Environmental groups are trusted and mistrusted in almost equal measure (31% trust, 28% not trust), while scientists working for major companies are treated warily (20% trust, 42% not trust).

People, whether within groups or as individuals, have different perceptions of risk. Most experts' view of risk is shaped by the collection and analysis of data, the assessment of probability and the evaluation of possibilities. However, even those

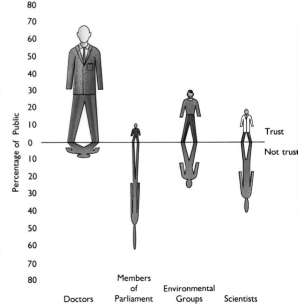

Figure 6.1
Results of a 1985 MORI opinion poll showing the degree of public trust in selected professional groups.

supposedly objective methods of risk assessment can be shaped by the subjective nature of the inputs and interpretation of outputs[245]. Scientists too are influenced by background, training and dominance of current models[246]. Members of the public often have a different perception of the adverse event than do experts who try to use objective methods of risk estimation[247]. Because hard data may be lacking, objective estimation of risk is sometimes able to deal only with human mortality, whereas public perception of a pollution incident, for example, takes into account wider consequences such as morbidity, harm to wildlife, and loss of amenity[248]. An example is the perception of the risk of lead poisoning in children. Some scientists may base their estimates of risk upon data on a few deaths and records of diagnosed cases of acute lead intoxication. However, the public perception is of risk to childrens' intelligence and behaviour over the long term, which is harder to evaluate, but of sufficient concern for the Government's Working Party on Inorganic Contaminants in Food to have reported that for bottle-fed infants, weekly intake of lead must not exceed 15 μg l^{-1}. Allowing for exposure to lead from dust and the air, this means that the level of lead in the water used to make up the feed must not exceed 10 μg l^{-1} on average. The current UK legal standard is 50 μg l^{-1} [61].

Research suggests that public perception of risk bears little relation to the degree of risk when expressed as a mathematical probability, but depends on several of other factors, such as whether the taking of risks is voluntary or involuntary, whether the hazards affect individuals or the whole of society, whether damage occurs in the short- or long-term, and whether the adverse event affects a small or large number of people[242]. Pesticides are an obvious focus for public concern because these are chemicals that are used specifically for their toxicity towards living organisms; they are purposely released into the environment; and humans are unavoidably exposed to pesticide residues in the food they eat and the water they drink. The amount of these residues may depend on the assiduity with which, for example, water is treated; but some residue, however small, is essentially inevitable.

In a 1980 survey in the USA[247] four groups of people (League of Women Voters, college students, active club members and scientific experts) were asked to rank 30 different activities and technologies in order of risk. It is apparent from this survey (Table 6.1) that pesticides are a class of chemicals that are perceived as a high risk, not only among members of the public but also by scientific experts. That perceived risk does not always match actual risk is clear from the views of college students, where pesticides were ranked higher than motor vehicles and motor cycles.

Scientific research can provide a framework for decisions on risk management, but as the Royal Commission on Environmental Pollution concluded, it is not the only factor that helps to determine policy[248]. Public opinion, where it can be reliably gauged, is another important factor. In forming its opinions the public is heavily influenced by what it learns from the media and the way in which issues are presented. There have been examples of relatively small risks becoming magnified when the public have seen major hazards where there was little evidence

	League of Women Voters	College students	Active Club members	Experts
Nuclear power	1	1	8	20
Motor vehicles	2	5	3	1
Handguns	3	2	1	4
Smoking	4	3	4	2
Motorcycles	5	6	2	6
Alcoholic beverages	6	7	5	3
General (private) aviation	7	15	11	12
Police work	8	8	7	17
Pesticides	9	4	15	8
Surgery	10	11	9	5
Fire fighting	11	10	6	18
Large construction	12	14	13	13
Hunting	13	18	10	23
Spray cans	14	13	23	26
Mountain climbing	15	22	12	29
Bicycles	16	24	14	15
Commercial aviation	17	16	18	16
Electric power (non-nuclear)	18	19	19	9
Swimming	19	30	17	10
Contraceptives	20	9	22	11
Skiing	21	25	16	30
X-rays	22	17	24	7
High school and college football	23	26	21	27
Railroads	24	23	20	19
Food preservatives	25	12	28	14
Food colouring	26	20	30	21
Power mowers	27	28	25	28
Prescription antibiotics	28	21	26	24
Home appliances	29	27	27	22
Vaccinations	30	29	29	25

Table 6.1
**Ranking of activities and technologies in order of risk
(1 = highest risk)**

of real potential damage. This does not mean that the strength of public opinion in these circumstances is not a valid reason for governments to take action, since that is a matter for political judgement. Commercial manufacturers and retailers are also keenly aware that public perceptions, regardless of their objective accuracy, can have very real economic consequences to which they must respond[249]: the case of consumer demand for additive-free food is a good example.

ASSESSMENT METHODS: TOXICOLOGY AND EPIDEMIOLOGY

The assessment of risk of chemical substances, including pesticides, is the concern of the toxicologist. The most commonly accepted definition of toxicology – the science that studies the adverse effects of chemicals on living organisms and assesses the probability of their occurrence – clearly indicates that risk assessment is an integral component of the discipline. A wider definition of toxicology would be 'the study and safety evaluation of chemicals and the manner in which they gain entry into living organisms, their effects from the molecular structure to the population level and the protective responses that they induce'[250]. There are two ways in which the potential adverse effects of pesticides on human health can be evaluated: tests on laboratory animals, micro-organisms and cultured cells; and human epidemiology studies.

The interface between epidemiology and toxicology is often fraught, the toxicologist arguing that the tighter specification of animal studies, and the absence of the social and environmental factors that confuse the issue in human studies, tempts one to regard the animal studies as more informative. However, the epidemiologist's view is that the greater relevance of the species, and the greater relevance of the dose in that species, makes the epidemiological data more informative[244]. These differences become most apparent when considering carcinogens. It is both unethical and impractical to expose humans to compounds and wait and see if cancers occur. Animal studies are subject to regulations, Good Laboratory Practice (GLP). A rodent cancer bioassay can be completed within 3 years (animal life span = 2 years, pathological and quantitative analyses up to 1 year), and therefore toxicology may be described as a prospective study while epidemiology is largely retrospective.

With human mortality studies one literally has to sit and wait for the subject to die (apart from cancer cases that are referred to a cancer registry). The cause of death can sometimes be totally unrelated to the study, for example accident, suicide or murder (Table 6.2). Finally, one is then reliant upon medical personnel to give an unbiased death certificate, which is then International Cause of Death (ICD) coded by a nosologist. The vital status of a human subject that is included in an epidemiology study is generally gauged by an initial questionnaire, and the smoking/drinking habits taken on trust. A new employee in a factory would be unlikely to admit to chronic and excessive alcohol use and/or smoking. The external influences of his social activities could give rise to misleading data if indeed he were to die from lung cancer, and the study was investigating the effects of compound 'x' on the incidence of respiratory cancer in his factory. Such a response related to a population could result in misleading bias. However, compare this example

Smoking 10 cigarettes a day	one in 200
All natural causes, age 40	one in 850
Any kind of violence or poisoning	one in 3300
Influenza	one in 5000
Accident on the road	one in 8000
Leukaemia	one in 12500
Playing soccer	one in 25000
Accident at home	one in 26000
Accident at work	one in 43500
Radiation working in radiation industry	one in 57000
Homicide	one in 100000
Accident on railway	one in 500000
Hit by lightning	one in 10000000
Release of radiation from nearby nuclear power station	one in 10000000

Table 6.2
Risk of an individual dying in any one year from various causes

Source: Living with Risk. BMA, 1990

to a rat study where external influences and socio-economic factors are nil and health status on entry into the study is guaranteed. Also the historical control data provides assurance of detecting genuine compound-related effects. One can be confident of minimal compounding factors and single compound exposures in toxicology studies, but not in epidemiology studies.

A further difference between the two types of studies is in the pattern and level of exposure. Both animal and human studies may be investigating the same chemical, but the means to the end is quite different. Suppose the pesticide in question was used in spraying maize. Two potential human groups to study would be:

1 *applicators*, having exposure occasionally to significant amounts, then periods of no exposure at all, with concurrent exposure to other chemicals.
2 *The general population*, who may consume the produce on average twice a week, taking in only very small amounts as a food contaminant.

Not only is the pattern and level of exposure different for the two groups of humans potentially at risk, but the routes of exposure are dissimilar. The applicators are exposed mainly through dermal absorption (99%: inhalation and oral routes being negligible), but to more than one pesticide, while the general population is exposed by the oral route (to presumably many chemicals including several pesticides at extremely small doses).

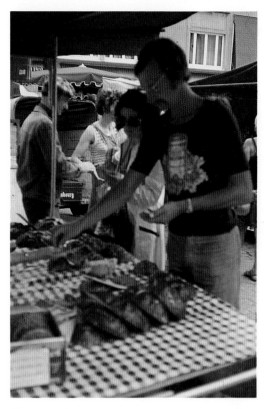

The general population may consume produce that has been treated with pesticides at various stages in its production.

Thus epidemiology of necessity studies populations of great genetic heterogenicity, of wide age distribution (at least within 18–65 years for industrial working age range and lifetime for environmental agents). The study populations are exposed intermittently to largely unknown concentrations of the toxicant of interest, by an ill-defined combination of routes, almost never in isolation, for which outcomes or effects are rarely determinable or even definable in the precise terms that are demanded of animal studies[251].

Animal tests, even when clearly positive, are inherently less useful than definitive well-designed epidemiological studies. This is because humans may not respond to a substance in the same way as an animal does and *vice versa*. Some chemicals not carcinogenic in animals (arsenic and phenacetin, for instance) are carcinogenic in humans. 2-Naphthylamine is a bladder carcinogen in humans and dogs, but not in mice, rats, guinea pigs and rabbits. However, the chemical can cause tumours in other sites in animals, principally the liver in rodents[252]. Furthermore, there is increasing evidence that it is genotoxic carcinogens that add most to the cancer burden in man. Identification of these genotoxic carcinogens and subsequent lowering of exposure will remain the main goal for primary cancer prevention in man[253,254].

In addition, laboratory exposures of animals to pesticides are not necessarily the same as under field conditions, where humans will often be exposed to a range of pesticides at one time, in varying climatic conditions. Laboratory tests are designed to cause a response in animals, from which safety margins can be calculated from known or predicted human exposure. The skill

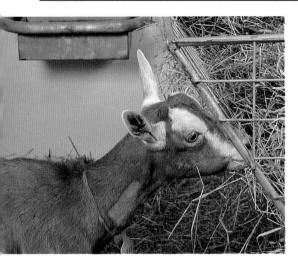

Biotransformation of pesticides in the food chain may alter their toxic potential. Studies in human food producing animals such as cattle, pigs and goats are conducted to assess these risks.

of the toxicologist is in identifying the most appropriate animal models that are relevant to humans.

A review[255] examining the emphasis placed on animal tests as predictors of carcinogenicity found that no systematic studies had been conducted to compare the results of cancer-predicting tests. There was a wide variance in the accuracy of some tests. Some bioassays such as the Ames test might be 90% accurate in testing some chemical groups; but with others, for instance those containing DDT and dieldrin, a very low level of accuracy in identifying mutagens was achieved. The Ames test will identify chemicals that damage DNA (Deoxyribonucleic acid, the main carrier of genetic information), but other tests are needed for carcinogens that act in other ways[256]. Available data suggest that those substances displaying carcinogenic properties in humans can generally be shown to produce similar effects in animals. However, that animal data reflect the humans data and *vice versa* for the majority of known human carcinogens is not an adequately reliable indicator for hazard.

In a widely publicized article published in 1987, Ames and his colleagues[257] challenged the validity of animal carcinogenicity data for estimation of risk to humans. Animal bioassays and *in vitro* studies can provide clues as to which carcinogens and mutagens might be contributing to human cancer. However, extrapolation from the results of rodent cancer tests (done at very high doses) to effects on humans (exposed to low doses) is extremely difficult. There is, argued the authors, little sound scientific basis for this type of extrapolation, in part due to our lack of knowledge about the mechanisms of cancer induction. Possible hazards to humans from a variety of rodent carcinogens (including the pesticides DDT and EDB) were ranked by an index that relates the potency of each carcinogen in rodents to the level of exposure in humans. According to Ames and his colleagues, the carcinogenic hazards of these levels of exposure to pesticide residues are likely to be of minimum concern to human health, compared with background levels of 'natural substances' such as aflatoxin in peanuts and ethyl alcohol. However, as Epstein and Schwartz stated in their 1988 rejoinder to Ames 'the existence of natural hazards clearly does not absolve industry and government from the responsibility of controlling industrial hazards'[258].

Human epidemiological studies suffer from the self-evident limitation that they are usually carried out retrospectively, and the data can be hard to obtain or of limited usefulness. Because of these limitations the determination of the potential to cause carcinogenic and other adverse effects does usually come from the results of laboratory animal tests.

DATA COLLECTION

Information is the lifeblood of epidemiology. As a joint report by the BMA and the Faculty of Community Medicine stated in 1979, 'all community physicians require ready access to information services. . . . It is no more possible to practise community medicine effectively in the absence of such supporting skills than to practise clinical medicine acceptably in the absence of laboratory and radiological facilities'[259]. Ultimately, epidemiology is concerned with the collection and analysis of data, and the presentation of that data as meaningful information[260–262].

Despite the importance of accurate information gathering to epidemiological research, there has been criticism of the lack of data available, particularly on the long-term effects of pesticides. The Report of the Chairman of the House of Commons Agriculture Committee on the effects of pesticides on human health[2] expressed concern that 'none of the government agencies involved with pesticides seems to have made *any* serious attempt to gather data on the chronic effects of pesticides on human health.' There are several data collection bodies, but none of these seem to be able to provide much useful information on the long-term health effects. The Health and Safety Executive admitted to the Committee that it only collects data on acute cases: 'the known statistics on poisoning, ill health and disease in agriculture do not allow us to form any judgement on illness resulting from chronic exposure.' Similarly, MAFF indicated that they have no system for routinely monitoring any possible chronic effects caused by pesticide use, or of determining the extent to which they occur. The Advisory Committee on Pesticides is charged with responding to data received rather than acting as an initiator of enquiries.

Neither NHS hospitals nor the National Poisons Unit (NPU) are in a position to make much more of a contribution to epidemiological research. The National Poisons Information Service (NPIS) and the regional centres were established to deal with the problems of acute poisoning, and few enquiries from medical practitioners relate to chronic effects[263]. In evidence to the Agriculture Committee, the NPIS expressed concern about under-reporting and claimed that doctors' failure to recognize symptoms and signs of acute poisoning may be one reason for under-reporting. It was estimated that centres in the UK receive enquiries on only about 50% of suspected poisonings seen by general medical practitioners. Moreover, it was suggested that many members of the public who are exposed to agrochemicals do not seek medical attention[2].

Other data collection bodies include the Medical Research Council, which is supporting research into the long-term effects of worker exposure to phenoxy herbicides, although this research does not have a high priority. Some of the larger pesticide manufacturing companies have themselves carried out regular monitoring of their employees for many years and these data are regularly scanned for health trends. However, extrapolation of data from a human population in a carefully controlled manufacturing environment to the general public – including the very young and old, the sick, pregnant women and so on – is fraught with problems.

The conclusion drawn from this by the Chairman of the Agriculture Committee was that: 'in view of the undoubted public concern about possible chronic health effects of pesticide use, we find this lack of epidemiological research quite unsatisfactory and urge greater efforts to be made in this area by the responsible public authorities'[2].

SETTING LIMITS

In the past, great weight has been attached to the acute toxicity of pesticides as indicated by animal tests relating to LD_{50} research. LD_{50} stands for the dose administered to a group of animals that causes the death (hence LD, lethal dose) of 50% of those animals. LD_{50} is adjusted to take account of body weight. The acute effects of pesticides should not be underestimated. In developing countries one of the most serious dangers to operators (and to a lesser extent to the wider public) comes from acute pesticide poisoning.

However, in developed countries, a greater perceived risk comes from long-term exposure, whether in the work setting or from residues in food and water. For some pesticides there are occupational threshold limits known as Threshold Limit Values (TLVs) or Occupational Exposure Limits (OELs). TLVs do not exist for many pesticides and, when they do, the values can differ substantially from one country to another.

If a pesticide is applied in accordance with good agricultural practice, any residue left in the crop should not exceed what is known as the Maximum Residue Level (MRL). These statutory levels are set for individual pesticides in individual or groups of foods as they leave the farm gate. The aim is to keep residues as low as possible, and therefore the existence of a statutory level does not mean that higher levels would necessarily give rise to toxic effects in humans, because the safety margins applied are so large.

In the UK, statutory controls on pesticide residues in food were introduced for the first time in 1988 when the Government set legally enforceable MRLs for 62 pesticides used in 'the most important fruit and vegetable components of the average national diet.' The legislation, the Pesticides (Maximum Residue Level in Food Regulations) 1988, comes under Part III of the Food and Environment Protection Act 1985. The MRL is expressed as milligrams of the residue per kilogram of the commodity. But when the UK regulations came into force in January 1989 they omitted 31 MRLs which the Government had proposed to set the previous April. In a further 24 cases, the regulations set statutory MRLs which were less stringent than had been proposed by the Government in April. The omission included MRLs for certain pesticides in celery, potatoes and lettuce.

According to the Government report, published in 1987, the treatment of protected crops of cos and butterhead lettuce at the minimum UK-recommended harvest interval of 7 days resulted in residues of iprodione (a fungicide) which 'tended to exceed' the non-statutory MRL recommended by the FAO/WHO Codex Alimentarius Commission[264]. Similarly, this 1987 report also mentioned that residues of dimethoate (an insecticide) in 'protected crop' lettuces also 'tended to exceed' the Codex MRL.

The Government also back-tracked on proposals to set statutory MRLs for ethylene bis-dithiocarbamates (a class of fungicides, also called EBDCs) on lettuce and celery. In January 1990, the Government's Advisory Committee on Pesticides reported that residues of dithiocarbamates 'could and should be reduced'. There are still no statutory MRLs for EBDCs as proposed by the Government in April 1988.

The toxicological significance of any residue is assessed through long-term studies in animals to establish the highest dose of pesticide, in milligrams per kilogram of body weight, at which no effect on health is observed. The studies have to cover possible production of cancers of various types, birth and inheritance defects as well as effects on the nervous and reproductive systems. The 'no observable effect' level in the most sensitive test species is used to set the Acceptable Daily Intake (ADI) in man. The ADI is the amount of a pesticide that can be ingested every day throughout a person's life with the practical certainty, based on the known facts, that no harm will result. For a given pesticide the MRL must be set at a level such that the consumer does not receive more than the ADI. The government samples food for residues on both individual product and total diet bases, taking into account variations in dietary habits within the population, with the aim of ensuring that consumers are not exposed to residues that exceed the ADI. Both MRLs and ADIs are allocated to individual pesticides by WHO and are harmonized throughout the world by the Codex Alimentarius Commission of the UN which is supported by 130 countries.

Maximum Admissible Concentrations (MACs) for drinking water were set by the EEC in its 1980 *Directive on Drinking Water Quality*, which came into force in 1985. The MAC for pesticides is $0.1 \, \mu g \, l^{-1}$ (0.1 parts per billion) for individual pesticides and $0.5 \, \mu g \, l^{-1}$ (0.5 parts per billion) for total pesticides, irrespective of their individual toxicity. This compares with 50 parts per billion (ppb) each for arsenic, cyanides and lead in running water, and one part per billion for mercury.

The fact that pesticides are found in water and food at all are seen by some as a cause for concern, but in most cases the concentrations are so low that they are usually measured in parts per billion. The rate of advance in analytical techniques over the past few years means that it is now possible to measure in parts per trillion, and occasionally per quadrillion. At the current rate of advance, it will be possible to measure a few molecules in the not too distant future. It may appear to the consumer that there is a growing problem with concentrations of pesticides, simply by virtue of the fact that today's sophisticated diagnostic methods enables us to detect pesticides at levels that were previously too small to trace. This is just one of the paradoxes of public perceptions of risk with regard to pesticide exposure.

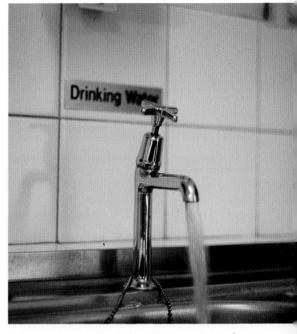

Concern about the quality of drinking water has led to recent increases in consumption of bottled water.

RISKS TO CONSUMERS AND THE GENERAL PUBLIC

Food

The wider public are exposed to pesticides largely through the food they eat and the water they drink. This is undoubtedly a cause of major public concern, part of a general crisis of confidence in the wholesomeness of food. The general public fears not only pesticides, but also listeriosis and salmonella poisoning, food additives, hormones and antibiotics in meat,

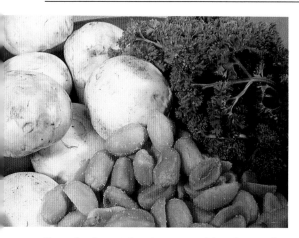

Some foods contain minute quantities of naturally occurring toxins.

dioxin in milk cartons, lead soldered food cans and food irradiation: the list goes on. Food should be the least of our worries: smoking a pack of 20 cigarettes a day increases a woman's risk of cancer 14-fold; even radon in the soil poses a cancer risk of one in 1000. But risk has its own psychology. Smoking is voluntary; radon is natural and ranting at nature does nobody any good. Since food is supposed to be pure and safe, people are outraged if it poses any risk at all. It has to be remembered that some foods contain minute quantities of naturally occurring toxins. For example, mushrooms contain hydrazines, peanuts aflatoxins, parsley psoralen, and rhubarb oxalic acid.

It is difficult to open a newspaper or magazine nowadays, here and in the USA, without reading another article about the hazards of the family diet. A survey carried out by the Consumers Association in 1988 asked people what they thought about the treatment of fruit and vegetables with pesticides. Seventy-four per cent of respondents were of the opinion that 'some chemical treatment residues on fresh fruit and vegetables are dangerous to health', 62% of respondents were 'prepared to pay more for food produced without chemicals' and 79% felt that 'fresh fruit and vegetables should be labelled to show which chemical treatments have been used'. A further survey in February 1990 found that half the people who bought organic food thought it was better for their health, and one in six thought it was better for the environment.

The American public feels much the same. A Gallup poll published in *Newsweek* in March 1989 showed that 38% of Americans are 'more worried that the food they eat may be contaminated with pesticides and other toxic chemicals', and 73% felt that less pesticide should be used even if this meant higher prices. Supermarkets here and in the USA are reporting a 'panic for organic'. Only a tiny proportion (perhaps 1%) of agricultural land is devoted to production of crops without the use of agricultural chemicals and it will take years to convert more to organic production.

Do consumers have any reason to worry? The Government maintains that current standards are now sufficiently rigorous for there to be no risk to the general public from residues in food. As described in the previous section (*Setting Limits*), statutory controls on pesticide residues in food were introduced for the first time in 1988 with the setting of MRLs for 62 pesticides used in the most important fruit and vegetable components of the average national diet. Coordination of the monitoring of pesticide residues is the responsibility of the MAFF Working Party on Pesticide Residues. The Working Party oversees the monitoring of residue levels both in home-produced and imported food, and in human tissues, wildlife and the environment. A rolling programme of surveys on major food commodity groups (that is, fruit and vegetables, cereals and animal products) has been supplemented with a programme of continuous monitoring of three major components in the national diet (bread, milk and potatoes). A survey of retail fruit and vegetables was carried out in 1982–86, and a survey of retail animal products in 1985–88. The results of these surveys have been published in three reports – the most recent, for the period 1985–88, published in 1989[265].

The Report of the Working Party on Pesticide Residues is by

far the most comprehensive survey of pesticide residues in our diet. The most recent report contains the results of the British Total Diet Study for 1984–85: a survey of foodstuffs purchased fortnightly from population centres throughout Britain.

The survey of retail animal products in 1985-88 was the first detailed study of the topic. The most commonly detected residues were pp'DDE, a metabolite of DDT, and gamma-HCH, a form of hexachlorocylcohexane. Residues were most commonly found in lamb, and the explanation is thought to be the use of DDT and HCH in sheep dips. Following the withdrawal of these products in sheep dips from January 1985 levels were observed to fall, but HCH was still detectable in 10% of samples of lamb in 1986. All samples of processed pork and poultry from China were found to contain organochlorine residues, in most cases exceeding the MRL.

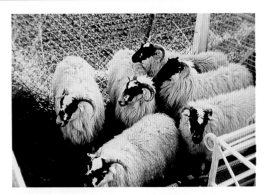

A survey of retail animal products found that residues in lamb may have come from sheep dips.

Thirty-seven out of 67 samples of potatoes analysed in the survey contained residues of tecnazene at levels at or in excess of the EC MRL of 1 mg kg^{-1}. Tecnazene is used as a fungicide and sprout inhibitor. Aware of the level of public concern and of how this might affect demand for their products, Marks and Spencer and Sainsbury carried out their own checks on potatoes and other fruit and vegetables, rejecting those containing unacceptable levels of tecnazene. Tecnazene was one of the major concerns of a confidential MAFF report on pesticide residues[40] leaked to Friends of the Earth in August 1988, and subsequently published. This report by the Residues Sub-Group of the Government's Research Consultative Committee stated that leafy vegetables and root crops 'are normally treated with fungicides for protection against storage diseases. Methods of application are fairly crude and more work is needed to determine the uniformity of fungicide distribution in relation to the permitted average residue levels'[40]. The report concluded that, in consequence, 'the levels of pesticide residues on stored produce leaving the farm gate can vary considerably from batch to batch'. The WHO Codex Committee recommended an MRL of 10 mg kg^{-1} for tecnazene.

The Sub-Group also noted 'concern' about residues in immature vegetables and reported that all the data supplied in application for approvals related to 'full-term crops', despite the large market for baby beetroot and carrots. Similarly, the report recommended that 'studies should be undertaken to investigate the implications for residues especially where the crop is grown in peat blocks treated with pesticide'. Some of the assumptions about 'healthy' food were challenged by the Sub-Group's other findings. They report that 'there remains a need for information about the fate of residues in bran during processing into bran-based products'[40].

The report criticized the 'bucket and shovel' method of applying pesticides to potatoes and other stored crops. This revelation is causing some people to question whether jacket potatoes really are better for you. In addition to tecnazene, potatoes imported from Cyprus have been found to contain residues of pirimiphos-methyl.

That a high-fibre diet is not entirely free of health risks was further highlighted in the Residues Sub-Committee report, which expressed concern over pesticide residues in bran, the outer layer of cereal which remains in wholemeal breads and

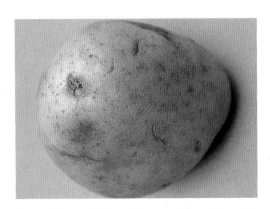

Most of the pesticide residue in potatoes is found in the skin.

Further information is needed concerning the effect of malting and brewing processes on residues in barley and other cereals.

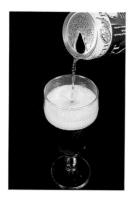

WHITE FLOUR; contains 30% of original residue on whole grain

WHOLEMEAL FLOUR; contains 60% of original residue on whole grain

BRAN; contains 3 to 4 times the amount of residue than that of whole grain

Figure 6.2
Bran has been found to be contaminated at levels 3–4 times that of the whole grain. White flour contains much less residue.

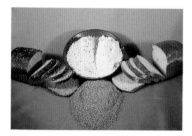

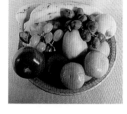

Pesticide residues in fruit are often measured in the skin only.

pastas. As with potatoes, the pesticides implicated are those used to prevent insect and fungal damage to grain during movement or storage. The Sub-Group stated that:

'Stored produce may also be subjected to repeated pesticide treatment or admixed with freshly treated produce introduced later into the storage container. Information is needed also, concerning the effect of malting and brewing processes on residues of organophosphorus insecticides in barley and other cereals. These data are required in order to evaluate exposure of the consumer to residues in retail products as a result of pesticide application to raw cereals.'[40]

In other words, beer may provide a surprising, added kick.

The Sub-Committee saw a need for greater monitoring of pesticide residues in stored foods, as well as the need for more information on the effects of malting and brewing processes on residues of organophosphorus insecticides in barley and on other cereals. At the same time a research review by the Home Grown Cereals Authority drew attention to the degradation of pesticides during milling and the possibility of pesticides 'bonding' with cereals making them difficult to detect or remove[266].

This review noted that fewer than 600 samples of UK home-grown wheat were reported as having been analysed for pesticide residues since 1970. The majority of samples were examined for organophosphorus pesticides only. A significant number of the samples analysed contained residues, but only a few were in excess of the MRL. It is surprising that there are no analytical data on pyrethroid residues, nor on cereals other than wheat, and there is an urgent need to fill these gaps in our knowledge. It may be, from the relatively limited data available, that we are almost certainly underestimating the level and range of pesticide contamination in grain. This is particularly important as very little loss of residues takes place during the milling of grain to produce flour and, although white flour contains only about 30% of the original residue, wholemeal flour contains at least twice this amount. Pure bran, however, because of its position on the outside of the grain, has been found to be contaminated at levels three or four times that of the whole grain (Figure 6.2). When baked into bread, both white and wholemeal flours may have reduced contamination levels of up to 50%. All these problems may arise from the fact that, although grain at harvest may be relatively uncontaminated with residues, it can be treated several times with pesticide, usually organophosphate, during storage[266].

Although bread is not the staple food that it once was, these findings have considerable importance in relation to dietary residues, particularly with regard to the increasing trend towards the consumption of wholemeal grain products.

Another problem concerns the monitoring of pesticide residues in fruit. The Sub-Group reported that: 'In most cases the levels of residues of post-harvest fungicides and anti-oxidants used on some fruits have been measured in the skin only but recent work indicates that, in certain cases, pesticides penetrate into the flesh of the fruit'.

Consequently, residue levels are probably generally diluted so that the concentrations in the flesh of the fruit may fall below levels that can be determined using current procedures. However, since the whole fruit is consumed, the total amount of pesticide in the fruit could be significantly more than that previously thought to be confined to the peel tissues. As a result consumers may be exposed to higher dosages of these chemicals than has hitherto been suspected'[40].

The Sub-Group has also pointed out that about 80% of the UK apple and pear crop is held in long-term storage requiring some form of post-harvest chemical application. They stated that there was thus 'an urgent need to re-examine the reliability of existing data on residue levels'[40].

The Total Diet Study is surveying an average intake for people eating an average diet. It does not take into account the growing numbers of ethnic minority groups who follow a diet totally different from the national diet. They are inclined to eat imported foods, which may have been grown using pesticides prohibited in Britain. Another group at potential risk are vegetarians. They tend to eat much more fruit and vegetables than would be found in the national average diet and it is fair to assume that they ingest a higher level of pesticides. In addition, they tend to make use of beans and pulses as a source of protein, and most of these are imported. The 1984 Steering Group on Food Surveillance suggested that to overcome the problems associated with ethnic minority and vegetarian diets, a duplicate diet study be carried out.

In view of the increasing trend towards high fibre and other 'health foods' the Working Party on Pesticide Residues[265] in 1985 commenced a study on food available from health food shops. Samples of pulses, herbal teas, honey, peanut butter, and vegetable oils were analysed. Although bromomethane is one of the fungicides commonly applied to imported commodities, including nuts, very little residue data were available. A survey was therefore carried out comparing residues in nuts in health food shops with other retail outlets. There was little difference between them. Although some pesticide residues were detected (pirimiphos-methyl in lentils, the fungicide dichlofluanid in raspberry leaf tea, quintozene in mung beans and so on) these were not at a level to cause concern and, again, there was little difference in residue levels in samples obtained from health food shops as compared with other retail outlets.

One additional point relating to pesticide residues in food arises from food irradiation. The government's Research Consultative Committee Residues Sub-Group reported in 1988 that 'one area of concern was the irradiation of commodities which contained pesticide residues and associated inert substances and the possibility of these residues being transformed into more toxic radiolytic products.'

Water

Using modern analytical methods, water can be analysed for extremely low concentrations of pesticides (down to $0.05 \mu g \, l^{-1}$ in some cases). However, the presence of a pesticide in water, even at levels above the MAC, may not in itself present a health risk to the consumer. It is necessary to take into account the known toxicology of individual chemicals and to consider how widespread is the presence of the chemical before the risk can be properly assessed[267].

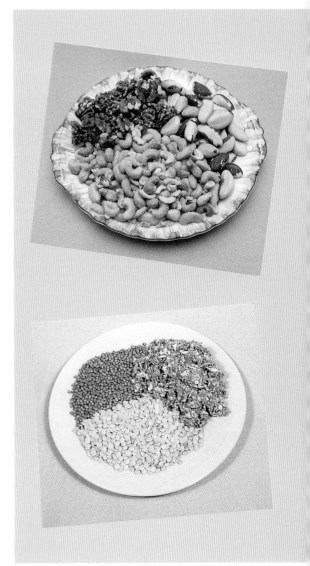

A greater awareness of nutrition and health has created a trend towards 'health foods'.

In August 1989 the results of an extensive survey of drinking water quality carried out by Friends of the Earth (FoE) was published. The ten water authorities of England and Wales were contacted by FoE in February 1989, asking for details of water samples that exceeded the EC's MAC for five types of chemicals: lead, aluminium, nitrates, pesticides and trihalomethanes (chemicals created by reactions involving chlorine used to treat tap water). The 28 privately owned water companies were also asked to supply the same details. According to FoE over two million people were found to be at risk from excessive concentrations of lead (over 50 µg l^{-1}). Two million people drink water containing more than the MAC of aluminium (200 µg l^{-1}). At least 1.7 million people consume water that exceeds the European limit for nitrate (50 µg l^{-1}).

FoE had earlier[50] identified 298 water supplies, and sources exceeding the MAC for pesticides. The published figures identified areas around London and the Home Counties, East Anglia and the East Midlands, Avon and Wiltshire, and North Yorkshire as having water supplies containing pesticide residues at levels higher than the MAC of 0.1 µg l^{-1} for individual pesticides, and 0.5 µg for all pesticides together. Among the pesticides detected at higher than MAC were 2,4-D around the Norwich area, atrazine and simazine in water from Graffham (which serves Bedford, Milton Keynes and Huntingdon), and 2,4,5-T in samples from the Anglian Water Authority.

The implications of mixtures of certain pesticides in drinking water, a situation highlighted by FoE's survey, has been considered by the World Health Organisation[268]. WHO stated that:

'The problem of exposure to any mixture of two or more of the herbicides . . . cannot be handled in isolation. . . . Drinking water may contain chemical residues of different types, including pesticides, other environmental contaminants, or micropollutants, many of which may as yet be unidentified. In addition, people are exposed to chemical substances by many other routes, which may also give rise to possible interactions. The complexity of the problem precludes simple answers.'[268]

WHO recommended that, 'the possible toxicological implications of such contamination should be assessed on a case-by-case basis . . . all available information on the toxicological properties of the individual substances must be collected in order to assess the hazard of each substance.'

RISKS TO CHILDREN

Our children rely on us to protect their health. They are too young to make assessments of the risks that surround them, or to take action as individuals or communities to reduce those risks. Their immaturity may also make them more vulnerable to toxic substances in their environment, including pesticides. Introducing its widely publicized report *Intolerable Risk*[269] the US Natural Resources Defense Council (NRDC), an environmental pressure group, claimed that experiments on laboratory animals have found the young to be more vulnerable than adults to the toxic effects of many chemicals, including a number of pesticides, due to their immature physiological systems. Studies suggest that the young of various species retain a far greater portion of a given dose of certain toxins than adults, because gastrointestinal absorption is increased and elimination decreased.

Studies noted in the NRDC report suggest also that there is a greater risk of developing cancer if exposure to carcinogens begins in infancy rather than later in life. The young have also been shown to be at greater risk from exposure to a number of neurotoxins, including neurotoxic pesticides. Young rats have been shown to be more susceptible than adults to the acute effects of 15 out of 16 organophosphate pesticides tested. In addition, experimental studies indicate that exposure to organophosphates and carbamate pesticides during the period of nervous system development in the neonate may alter neurological function and may cause subtle and long lasting neurobehavioural impairments[269].

Recently there has been considerable media coverage of the presence of pesticides in breastmilk and in apples. To many people the existence of toxic chemicals, in however minute a level, in these very symbols of healthy nurturing is particularly disturbing.

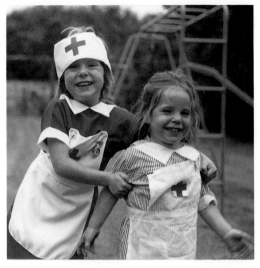

Children are too young to make assessments of the risks that surround them and are often more vulnerable than adults to toxic substances in the environment.

Breast Milk and Infant Feeding

Exposure to pesticides can begin in the very earliest days of a baby's life when feeding at the mother's breast. Even quite low exposure to pesticide residues can be reflected in human milk if these substances have a high degree of environmental and metabolic persistence, and are highly soluble in fat. In 1983 Jensen[270] summarized numerous studies reporting on levels of organochlorine residues in human milk from around the world. Use patterns of various pesticides were reflected in the residues in breast milk, with higher concentrations in Third World countries. Higher levels of DDT and aldrin were recorded in India, while dieldrin levels were highest in South American countries.

The WHO report *Chemical Contaminants in Food: Global Situation and Trends* states: 'The reported levels of pesticides and other contaminants in human milk at certain times result in estimated intakes by the breast fed infant that exceed toxicologically acceptable intake levels. Whether such intakes are detrimental to the child's progress in terms of physical or possibly mental development is not known.' However, there is a tendency to assume that infants are more susceptible than adults to toxic substances. Data to support this are not readily available: infants may be more, or less, susceptible. Moreover, the variation between adults is often greater than between children and adults[3].

Although the presence of pesticide residues in breast milk is an area for genuine concern, both because of the risk to infants and as an indicator of levels of pollution in the environment, it is important that women should not be led to believe that breast feeding is in some way less healthy than using formula feeds. The MAFF Working Party on Pesticide Residues carried out a survey in 1987 of infant foods (including rusks, tinned baby food, and formula milks). Two out of 50 samples of infant formula feeds contained low levels of organochlorine residues. The food that most widely contained pesticide residues was rusks. Eighteen out of 31 samples of rusks contained pirimiphos methyl at higher levels. In view of the reported concentration of pesticide residues in bran, it is surprising that the highest residue levels were not, in fact, found in wholemeal rusks. Three samples of cows' milk contained dieldrin at levels exceeding the EC MRL of 0.15 mg kg^{-1} fat. The Committee on Toxicity of Chemicals in Food, in considering the Working Party's report, were concerned that infants and young children drinking cows' milk with dieldrin at these concentrations could exceed the safety level of the ADI.

Apples and Alar

Since 1968 some red varieties of apple have been sprayed with daminozide, made by the Uniroyal Chemical Company under the trade name Alar. Daminozide is sprayed on apples at the blossom stage and is thereby incorporated into the fruit. It acts as a plant growth regulator, which keeps apples from dropping off the tree until they ripen. It has the effect also of improving colour and firmness, and extending shelf life. It is estimated to have been used until recently on at least 5% of apples in the USA, and on 7% of the British apple crop. It is used also on grapes, and has been used on hops in the UK. In the early 1980s the US Environmental Protection Agency (EPA) received several toxicity studies which indicated that a metabolite and breakdown product of daminozide called UDMH (unsymmetrical dimethylhydrazine) caused tumours in mice. UDMH forms when Alar is heated, as in the production of apple sauce or fruit juice. Daminozide also converts in the body to UDMH by a process of hydrolysis. The Alar case provides an important reminder of the way public perceptions of risk have a strong influence on risk management.

Alar, which was used on grape and apple crops, was withdrawn by the manufacturers following public concern about risks to children.

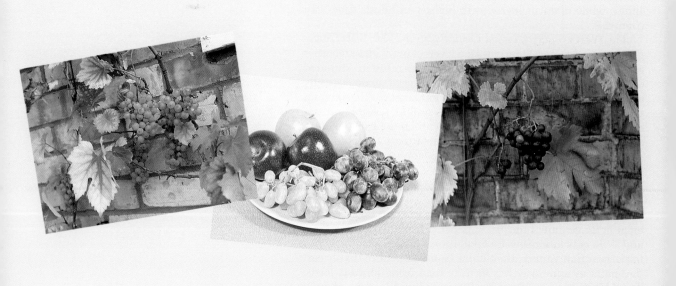

During February 1989 the EPA announced its intention to withdraw Alar within 18 months, commenting that the evidence was insuffucient for an immediate ban. At the end of the same month the US environmental pressure group the NRDC published the results of its 2-year study on the potential effects on children's health of some pesticides[269]. The study alleged that children under 6 years, who are likely to consume more fruit and fruit products than adults, are especially vulnerable to carcinogenic pesticides. On the basis of its assessment of risk, the NRDC stated that preschool children may develop cancer as a result of their exposure to eight of the most common pesticides (the fungicides captan, chlorothaoil, folpet and ethylene thiourea(ETU, the metabolite of mancozeb); acephate; the insecticides parathion and methyl parathion; and UDMH). The NRDC study cites UDMH as the most potent carcinogen, and predicts extra cancer risks of one in 1100. This is 900 times greater than the EPA's standard of acceptability which sets a lifetime risk of greater than one in a million to be unacceptable.

The NRDC report received considerable coverage on popular nationwide television programmes in the USA, which reach tens of millions of consumers[271,272]. Schools from coast to coast removed apples, apple juice and apple sauce from lunch menus. Organic food stores were overrun with demand for pesticide-free fruit. In a widely reported episode, an Oregon mother called out the Highway Patrol to apprehend her daughter's school bus; troopers stopped the bus and seized Sally's lunch box, which contained a bunch of grapes. Reaction in the UK was more temperate but there was still widespread coverage. A pressure group, Parents for Safe Food, was launched to campaign for more information to be made available to consumers on residues in food. Since launching the campaign, the group has received over 20000 letters, an eloquent testimony to a chord struck with many parents.

In February 1989, the US proposed a ban on Alar because of 'an inescapable and direct correlation between the use of Alar and the development of life-threatening tumours'. A month after indicating that it would recommend a ban the EPA reversed its advice, leaving parents confused as to whether the chemical poses a cancer risk or not. The California Department of Food and Agriculture condemned the NRDC report for lack of attention to science, and a statement from the US Surgeon General said, 'after reviewing the many studies of the possible harmful side-effects, officials of the Environmental Protection Agency, the Food and Drug Administration, Department of Agriculture and an independent scientific review board have each rejected recent claims that Americans face a public health threat from apples treated with Alar.' However, in an atmosphere of confusion, sales of apples and apple products fell dramatically. The manufacturers, Uniroyal, then voluntarily withdrew the pesticide from the US market[272].

The NRDC report[269] was examined by an independent reviewer, on behalf of the North American Chemicals Association[273]. It was heavily critical of the NRDC report, claiming that it was emotive and unscientific. While this may be expected of an industry-sponsored report, the review highlighted the fact that the NRDC report actually contained serious mathematical errors, which had led to an over-estimate of the risks, and that the basis of the report was scientifically unsound. The lesson contained herein is twofold. Firstly, the science of risk assessment is a new discipline and it is possible to draw very different conclusions from the same database. Secondly, unnecessary public anxiety can be caused by the misuse of science.

In the Alar case, the EPA vacillated between banning Alar and later stating that it was safe. While this is an example of the 'precautionary principle' in practice, it is clear that for this to be effective, objectivity and science are prerequisite.

In the UK, the Advisory Committee on Pesticides considered all available data on daminozide and concluded that there was no health risk. However, manufacturers were asked for the results of further tests as quickly as possible. These were received in September 1989, and the interim results were communicated for the first time by the Agriculture Minister, Baroness Trumpington. Mice given 'very high doses' of daminozide did develop lung and liver tumours; although no figures are given for these doses MAFF states that these were massive compared with any amounts likely to be encountered by humans. These preliminary results have been reported also to a Joint Meeting on Pesticide Residues of WHO and FAO, on which the UK is represented. This body has now decided that an ADI of 0.5 mg kg^{-1} could safely be set for daminozide. In December 1989 the Advisory Committee on Pesticides presented to ministers the final report on its review of daminozide. The Committee concluded that:

1 The safety factors for daminozide range from 4,000 to 6,000 times greater than the no-effect level in animals.
2 For UDMH the safety factors range from 150 to 1,000 times greater than the no-effect level.
3 Even for infants and children consuming the maximum quantities of apples and apple juice, subjected to the maximum treatment with daminozide, there is no risk from UDMH.

Although approvals for the use of products containing daminozide did not expire until 31 December 1990, the companies concerned made a commercial decision to withdraw the products for food related uses.

In a press release Uniroyal stated: 'We continue to believe that daminozide use on food crops does not pose a significant risk to public health.' The decision was made on commercial grounds because, 'even if further tests were successful, growers and the food industry would be very unlikely to come back to the product in any meaningful way.'

RISKS TO WILDLIFE AND THE ENVIRONMENT

Pesticides affect the health of living organisms in the same way as they do human health, either through direct contamination or through residues in food and water. They can also alter the numbers, distribution, and balance between species and so have important ecological effects. All species are affected: plants, fungi, bacteria, viruses, aquatic and other micro-organisms, insects, and larger forms of life such as fish, birds and mammals. The use of pesticides is just one aspect of modern

Pesticide users must consider the risks to all wildlife.

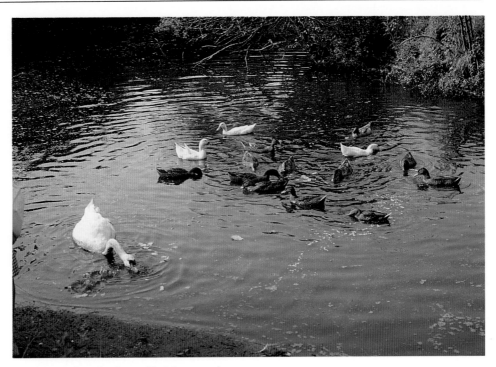

farming practice which has led to the erosion of habitats and food sources for a wide range of wildlife.

In 1955 the Advisory Committee on Poisonous Substances used in Agriculture and Food Storage (which later became the Advisory Committee on Pesticides) widened its terms of reference to allow consideration of the risks to wildlife. In 1959 a Wildlife Panel was set up. Under the Food and Environment Protection Act 1985, the need to safeguard the environment as well as human health received new emphasis. The Wildlife Panel continues to meet and produces periodic reports, now under the title of the Environmental Panel of the Advisory Committee on Pesticides.

The most recent report covers investigations of suspected poisoning of animals by pesticides in Great Britain 1985 to 1987[274]. The Wildlife Incident Investigation Scheme covers incidents involving vertebrate wildlife, companion animals (dogs, cats and so on) and honey-bees. Occasional cases of livestock poisoning are investigated, but these are also investigated independently by the MAFF Central Veterinary Laboratory. Between October 1985 and December 1986 a total of 558 incidents was investigated and 41% were shown to be associated with pesticides. During 1987 a further 624 incidents were investigated, with 35% attributable to pesticide poisoning. Among livestock and companion animals the average proportion of deaths caused by pesticides was 26%, but in honey-bees it was as much as 72%[275].

The MAFF investigations show that the largest cause of pesticide related mortality amongst wildlife is deliberate illegal abuse, generally involving poison baits in an attempt to kill predators. Although the range of pesticides used in this way is broad, it is dominated by three chemicals with minor approved uses (strychnine, alphachloralose, and mevinphos). The hazards to livestock and beneficial insects arise largely from

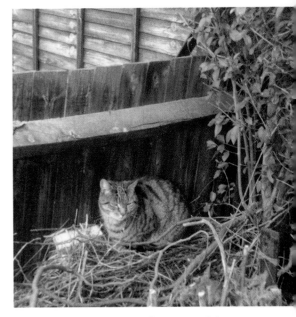

Man's companion animals such as cats and dogs are also susceptible to pesticide poisoning.

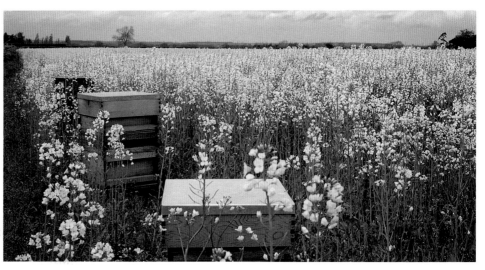

Harm to beneficial insects, such as honeybees, arises largely from careless handling of chemicals.

careless handling. For honey-bees the chief problem remains the use of triazophos on oilseed rape, partly through failure to observe the prescribed crop conditions in which spraying is permitted.

Although the Ministry of Agriculture monitoring shows that the majority of 'wildlife incidents' result from illegal use of pesticides, it is hard to see how this can be substantiated given the under-reporting of incidents, limited funds for testing of animal corpses, and general lack of research on the subject. There have been no major Government studies on the effects of pesticides on wildlife. The little information we have comes from the Working Party on Pesticide Residues, which in its third report[265] published the results of specific surveys of freshwater eels, wood-pigeons and wild rabbits.

There has been concern for some time about high levels of dieldrin in eels. It now appears that in addition to dieldrin, levels of DDT metabolites and HCH isomers were 'unexpectedly high' in a number of cases. Residues tend to be high in eels because of the high proportion of fat in their muscle tissues. The Department of Health regards dieldrin 0.07–0.1 mg kg^{-1} to be acceptable in fish. The MAFF sampling recorded levels ten times higher than this in a number of rivers, particularly those in Scotland. All approvals for DDT were revoked in October 1984, and approvals for dieldrin were revoked from the end of 1989. The Working Party expressed its concern that eels with high residue levels may present a potential threat to the long-term health of people who consume them in large quantities, to fish-eating birds, and to wild animals such as otters. More than 500 tonnes eels are harvested from British waters each year, and most are exported to West Germany and the Netherlands. Wood-pigeons were also surveyed for organochlorine residues, on the basis that as a sedentary species residues would be likely to reflect local exposures. Of 122 samples, DDT metabolites were found in 42% (three samples at above the EC MRL) and gamma-HCH in 41%. DDT levels appear to be decreasing, but the continuance of HCH levels is not adequately explained.

Pesticides affect wildlife in a variety of ways including: direct poisoning, food chain poisoning, and long-term health effects. *Direct poisoning* – Herbicides are generally less toxic to animals than other categories of pesticide, but have major effects on plants. However, some herbicides do have a direct poisoning effect. Fungicides can be toxic to wildlife, especially when used in seed dressings. Insecticides are by far the most toxic category of pesticides and their use has led to many wildlife incidents. In the 1970s the use of carbophenothion as a seed dressing in Britain led to the death of large numbers of greylag and pink footed geese and whooper swans which ate treated seed spilt in the fields. Its use as a seed dressing was subsequently banned in Scotland and restricted in the rest of the UK. The use of aldicarb for eelworm control in sugar beet areas has been responsible for the deaths of many bird species – gulls, lapwings, stone curlews and so on. Since its reformulation from a liquid to a granule there have been fewer reports of wildlife poisoning.

Food chain poisoning – Food chain poisoning occurs when creatures 'higher up' the food chain, such as birds of prey and foxes, feed on pesticide contaminated creatures such as smaller birds, fish, mice, rats and so on. In doing so these larger creatures accumulate pesticide residues in their own body fat, tissues and organs. Sometimes a lethal dose may be ingested; alternatively a sub-lethal dose can lead to poor fertility, susceptibility to disease and failure to thrive. Insecticides, particularly the persistent organochlorines like DDT and dieldrin, provide the clearest examples of food chain poisoning. In the 1960s, especially in cereal growing areas, populations of birds of prey such as peregrine falcons, sparrowhawks, and owls, as well as foxes and badgers, were reduced to very low levels from food poisoning by dieldrin[275,276]. Because they are persistent and fat soluble, organochlorine insecticides accumulated in the bodies of wild animals, and reached the greatest concentrations in predators. Different organochlorines affected populations in different ways. DDT-type compounds reduced reproductive rates, caused by shell-thinning and embryo deaths. The more toxic cyclodiene compounds (such as aldrin and dieldrin) increased the mortality rate in adult birds through direct toxic effects[277]. As the use of these chemicals has been progressively restricted, sparrowhawks and other birds of prey have gradually recovered in numbers, and spread back to the areas from which they had been eliminated. The numbers of foxes and badgers have also now returned to their former levels.

Long-term risks to wildlife – Organochlorine insecticides, like DDT, affect calcium metabolism in animals. Predatory birds, especially fish-eating species, accumulated sub-lethal doses of pesticide in body fat and tissue through the food chain. The main effect was to inhibit fertility and reproduction. In many predatory birds, the egg shells produced by contaminated birds were too thin due to lack of calcium, and broke in the nest before the young could hatch.

In addition to direct poisoning effects, pesticides can disrupt the ecological balance of wildlife. The spraying of hedgerows has led to a decline in many wild plants. Once common crop weeds, such as corn cockle and cornflower have all but gone. As once common weeds are killed off others, such as field pansy, move in to fill the gap, becoming major weeds in their own right. Pesticides have also acted to remove the food sources and habitats of a wide range of wildlife, resulting in a loss of the variety and richness of our environment.

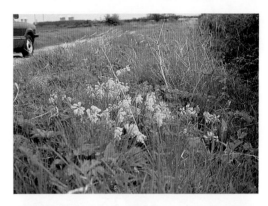

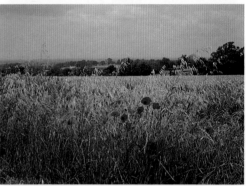

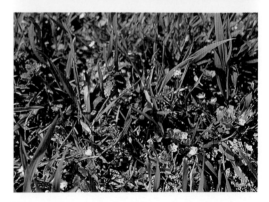

The use of pesticides has led to a decline in many wild plants.

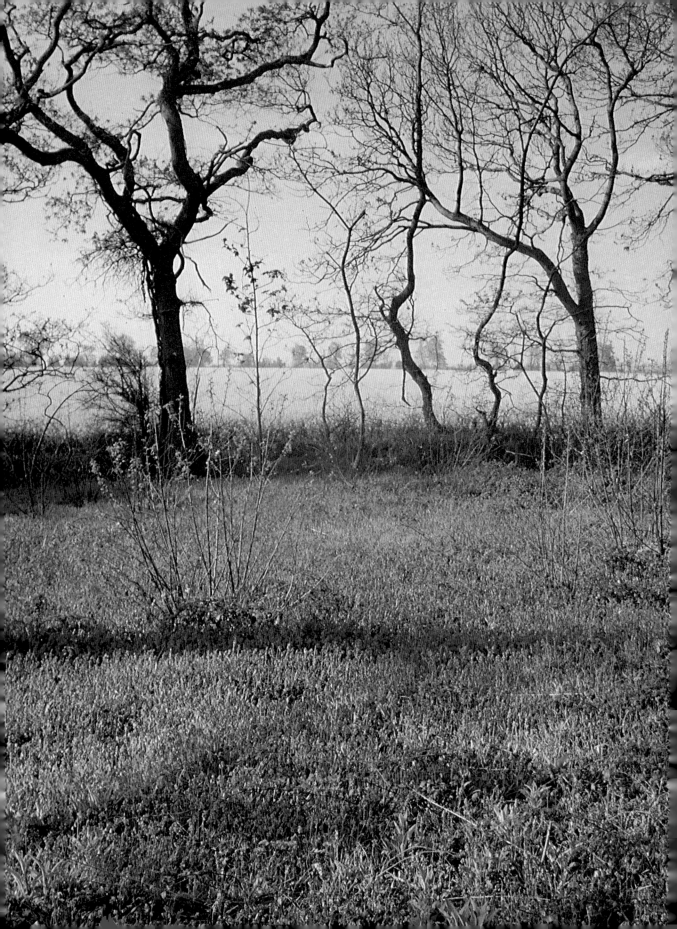

7 LAW AND ENFORCEMENT

STATUTES AND COMMON LAW

The laws covering the manufacture and use of pesticides can be confusing, both to those required to comply with them and for those seeking to use them to improve standards. There are at least two different sets of Regulations and Codes of Practice, based on different prevention and control philosophies, and with different legal duties and requirements. The responsibility for administering and enforcing the legislation is split between two different Government agencies: the Health and Safety Executive (HSE) and the Ministry of Agriculture Fisheries and Food (MAFF). The disposal of pesticides is a totally separate area, controlled by pollution legislation.

In addition to provision under statute law, health and safety at work and injury by pesticides in the wider community also falls under common law. Any injured party could, of course, seek redress through the civil courts in a claim for damages against a pesticide manufacturer or user. In practice this does not happen very often, and most problems are dealt with by statute law through the HSE and its enforcement officers, the HSE Agricultural Inspectorate. There are, however, few inspectors and only rare prosecutions. Fines for those convicted are often very low compared with the seriousness of the offence[83].

Figure 7.1
Six Government departments are involved in the process of approving pesticides for use.

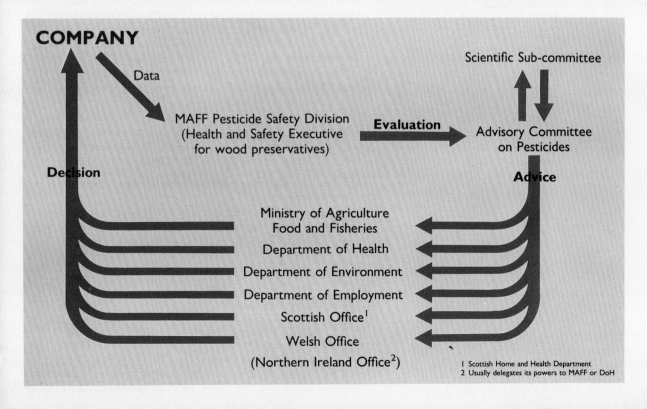

COMPANY

Data

Decision

MAFF Pesticide Safety Division
(Health and Safety Executive
for wood preservatives)

Evaluation

Scientific Sub-committee

Advisory Committee
on Pesticides

Advice

Ministry of Agriculture
Food and Fisheries
Department of Health
Department of Environment
Department of Employment
Scottish Office[1]
Welsh Office
(Northern Ireland Office[2])

1 Scottish Home and Health Department
2 Usually delegates its powers to MAFF or DoH

The current UK regulatory system for pesticides has three major areas of weakness:

1 The conflict of interest inherent in MAFF trying to regulate food production as well as pesticide safety.
2 The lack of enforcement of pesticide laws due to lack of health and safety inspectors and resources.
3 The lack of any legally empowered Safety Representative in agriculture, horticulture and forestry in line with other areas of industry.

Approval

Although the Advisory Committee on Pesticides has an important role in vetting pesticides, the main Secretariat for all agricultural and horticultural pesticides is MAFF (Figure 7.1). The HSE provides the Secretariat for wood preservatives and other non-agricultural uses. In practice this gives undue influence to the Ministry of Agriculture whose main role is food production, and there is, therefore, a conflict of interest inherent in MAFF having both these roles.

The US government, faced with a similar dilemma, removed pesticide control from the Agriculture Department and gave it to the Environmental Protection Agency (EPA). In the UK, given current regulatory arrangements, responsibility for pesticide approval should be transferred to HSE, away from MAFF.

Enforcement

Lack of enforcement of pesticide laws is a major weakness. The HSE has too few inspectors, especially Agricultural and Factory Inspectors, to carry out its general work on health and safety by making regular visits to factories, farms and other places, let alone cope with all the extra work generated by the new pesticide laws.

The main role for enforcing pesticide laws falls to the HSE Agricultural Inspectorate. Times between inspections of farms and horticultural premises have increased in the 1980s as the number of inspectors has been reduced. According to figures produced by the Institution of Professional and Managerial Staffs (IPMS), the trade union representing HSE Inspectors, visit frequencies have declined as follows:

1 Labour employing farms can expect a visit from an inspector every 5–8 years.
2 Self-employed farmers can run large farms and be major pesticide users. Their use of pesticides can pose a risk not only to themselves but to the public and environment. They can expect a routine visit, for any form of health and safety, once every 30 years.

Safety Representatives

British agricultural, horticultural and forestry workers have no legal right to appoint Safety Representatives to help protect their own health and safety and that of their colleagues, as well as helping to protect the public from dangers arising from work activities. Unlike other areas of industry, where safety representatives are permitted by law, agricultural and allied workers are exempted from the Safety Representatives and Safety Committee Regulations 1977 made under the Health and Safety at Work etc Act 1974. In other industries, under these Regulations, safety representatives have the following legal rights and powers:

1 To be nominated and appoint a trade union safety representative.
2 To be consulted by employers on health and safety matters, including risk assessments carried out under COSHH.
3 To inspect the workplace – on a quarterly basis as a minimum, and more often by agreement with management.
4 To receive information and assistance from management in carrying out their duties.
5 To require safety committees to be set up.
6 To receive time-off with pay to carry out their legal functions.
7 To receive paid time-off to undergo TUC or union approved health and safety training.

Safety Representatives are the backbone of trade union organizations on health and safety. In terms of safety, agriculture is the second or third most dangerous industry and one where accidents have increased by over 30% since the early 1980s. Agricultural workers similarly face a wide range of health problems from dusts and diseases as well as pesticides. This lack of legally appointed and empowered Safety Representatives in agriculture, forestry and horticulture is a major weakness in better implementation of pesticide laws. If the people who themselves face hazards are given legal powers to minimize those hazards, there will be an improvement not just in worker protection, but also in the quality of public and environmental health.

HEALTH AND SAFETY AT WORK ETC ACT 1974

The Health and Safety at Work etc Act 1974 is the main piece of health and safety legislation in the UK, and is one of the two major pieces of legislation covering pesticide use (the other being the Food and Environment Protection Act 1985). The Health and Safety at Work etc Act 1974 places duties on employers to safeguard their employees, and indeed members of the public, from hazards in the workplace. There are duties to provide and maintain safe premises and equipment; and to train, inform, instruct and supervise employees in health and safety matters. Duties extend to designers, suppliers and importers, to research and test machinery and substances for use at work, and to make available the results of those tests. The Safety Representative and Safety Committee Regulations 1977 give trade union safety representatives the right to investigate potential hazards in the workplace. However, agricultural and allied workers are exempted from these Regulations.

Specific Regulations under the 1974 Act are relevant to pesticide health and safety. These are as follows.

Control of Substances Hazardous to Health Regulations (COSHH) 1988

The COSHH Regulations are industry-wide measures which are controlled by the Health and Safety Executive. They provide for legal controls on all forms of substances hazardous to health – chemicals, dusts, fumes, fibres, micro-organisms and so on – in all work settings. Legal requirements for pesticide manufacture, formulation, storage and use are covered by these regulations, which lay down duties not only for employers but also for workers, self-employed people and contractors. The main COSHH Regulations are supported by Approved Codes of Practice. Those relevant to pesticides are the COSHH Approved Code of Practice for the Control of Exposure to Pesticides at Work, and COSHH Approved Code of Practice on Control of Exposure to Pesticide Fumigants at Work.

Health and Safety – Control of Industrial Major Accident Hazard Regulations 1984

These Regulations implement in the UK the EC Directive 82/501 on major accident hazards. They introduce requirements for the notification of sites where certain dangerous substances are involved and for the preparation of emergency plans.

Health and Safety – Classification, Packaging and Labelling of Dangerous Substances Regulations 1984

These Regulations cover chemical intermediates and technical pesticides, but pesticides that have been approved under the Control of Pesticides Regulations 1986 and are contained in packaging labelled in accordance with the approval are not included.

Health and Safety – Road Traffic (Carriage of Dangerous Substances in Packages etc) Regulations 1986

These Regulations set out the duties of operators and drivers of vehicles carrying dangerous substances in packages of more than a specified size.

FOOD AND ENVIRONMENT PROTECTION ACT 1985

The Food and Environment Protection Act 1985 (FEPA) is intended 'to protect the health of human beings, creatures and plants; to safeguard the environment; and to secure safe, efficient and humane methods of controlling pests'. It also seeks to 'make information about pesticides available to the public'. While the Health and Safety at Work etc Act is enforced by the Health and Safety Executive (HSE), FEPA is controlled by the Ministry of Agriculture, Fisheries and Food (MAFF). The Act regulates the import, sale, supply, storage, advertising and use of pesticides; sets maximum residue levels in food, crops and foodstuffs; provides for information to be made available to the public; and establishes the Advisory Committee on Pesticides. Flesh is put on the bare bones of the Act in the Control of Pesticides Regulations 1986.

Control of Pesticides Regulations 1986

These Regulations came into force in phases between October 1986 and January 1989, and now fully replace the old voluntary Pesticides Safety Precautions Scheme (PSPS). A summary of the Regulations, the stages of implementation and a glossary of key terminology has been produced as a useful factsheet by the British Agrochemicals Association[278]. The major provision is that no pesticide may be used commercially unless it has been given provisional or full approval on grounds of safety and efficacy by Ministers. The Regulations attempt also to answer the growing concern about aerial crop spraying, placing on users an obligation to 'take all reasonable precautions to protect the health of human beings, creatures and plants, to safeguard the environment, and in particular to avoid the pollution of water'.

Approvals – Since October 1986, only fully approved, provisionally approved, or experimental permit pesticides may be supplied, stored or used, and only provisionally or fully approved products may be sold. Approvals for industrial use of pesticides – approximately 10% of all approvals – are recommended by the HSE. Approvals for agricultural, horticultural, forestry and veterinary pesticides – the remaining 90% – are recommended by MAFF. All recommendations have to be approved by Ministers on the advice of the statutory Advisory Committee on Pesticides. Ministers can at any time review, revoke or suspend an approval. A full list of provisionally and fully approved pesticides is now available in published form from HMSO[279].

Competence – Sellers, suppliers, storers, and commercial users must be competent in their duties, and hold a recognized certificate of competence[280]. Commercial users must also have received adequate instruction and guidance in the safe, efficient and humane use of pesticides.

Advertising – Only provisionally or fully approved products may be advertised. All printed or broadcast advertisements must state the active ingredient.

Aerial spraying – Aerial applications are restricted to products that have specific approval for that purpose.

Pesticide residues in food – Where pesticides are used on food crops residues in food are covered by a separate set of regulations, the Pesticide (Maximum Residue Levels in Food) Regulations 1988. These introduce legal residue limits for some 60 pesticides, still only a minority of the pesticide active ingredients currently in use in the UK.

Storage – Work is now proceeding within MAFF on statutory codes of practice for the storage and disposal of all pesticides approved for agricultural use. A draft version is available from MAFF[281] giving guidance on the construction and siting of the store, transport requirements, and the supervision and training of staff.

PESTICIDES: CODE OF PRACTICE 1990

Pesticides: The Code of Practice for the Safe Use of Pesticides on Farms and Holdings in Great Britain (the 'Green Code') – prepared jointly by MAFF, the Health and Safety Commission and the Department of the Environment was published in May 1990. A combined Code of Practice under Part III of the Food and Environment Protection Act 1985 and the Health and Safety at Work etc Act 1974, it gives practical guidance to farmers, commercial crop growers and to those who provide advice or practical assistance, such as an agricultural contractor, to enable them to fulfil their legal obligation[282].

OTHER UK LEGISLATION

The Health and Safety at Work etc Act 1974 (with its Control of Substances Hazardous to Health Regulations 1988) and the Food and Environment Protection Act 1985 (with its Control of Pesticides Regulations 1986) form the main legislative framework controlling pesticides. Pesticides also feature in a lesser way in a number of other statutes.

Control of Pollution Act 1974

The effective disposal of old and withdrawn chemicals is a major problem. This Act regulates the disposal of surplus and waste pesticides (including those no longer approved for use) and empty pesticide containers. The Act, and the related Special Waste Regulations 1981, identifies a category of 'special waste' particularly hazardous to health. Most pesticides are classified as special waste, to be disposed of on special waste sites licensed and operated by the local authority. However, waste from premises used for agriculture within the meaning of the Agriculture Act 1947 is excluded from the definition of special waste, allowing farmers to dispose of pesticide waste on their own land. A Code of Good Agricultural Practice under the Control of Pollution Act covers pollution of water.

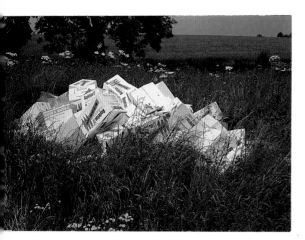

Pesticides which are not disposed of safely may pose a threat to health and the environment.

Consumer Protection Act 1987

This Act came into force on 1 March 1989, and seeks to impose stricter liability on producers of goods which are found to be defective, and which cause injury or loss. The Act does cover some foods, but specifically exempts agricultural produce unless it has undergone an industrial process. The law was passed in response to EC Directive 85/374 but in its exemption of many foods does not fulfil the directive, which exempts only those products that have undergone 'initial processing'. While including freezing, for example, the Act seems to exclude damage that might have been caused by pesticides[283]. This could lead to some interesting situations. If a farmer uses a pesticide that is later proved to cause injury and sells his produce at the farm gate (or to a wholesaler) the consumer has no remedy. But if he sells the produce to a canner, who then puts it through an 'industrial process', the consumer affected by pesticide contamination could hold the canner responsible. UK food laws can be seen to distinguish improperly between agricultural and industrial food processes, and provide a weak defence for the consumer against food residues and additives. The Food and Environment Protection Act 1985 was intended to meet this shortfall.

The Food Act 1984

This Act specifies the composition and labelling of food and includes reference to levels of pesticide residues.

Weights and Measures Act 1985

This Act makes requirements for fungicides and insecticides used as wood preservatives. No other pesticides are included, but where weights are given on containers they must comply with the Act.

Wildlife and Countryside Act 1981

This Act provides for the protection of certain species of British wildlife. In particular, all bats are now subject to special protection under the Act, and particular care must be taken when using wood preservatives. The effect of chemicals on wildlife is monitored by MAFF's Wildlife Incident Investigation Scheme, under which more than 200 cases of wildlife deaths that might be associated with pesticides are investigated in England and Wales each year.

The Animal (Cruel Poisons) Act 1962

This Act restricts the use of certain products as animal poisons.

The Animals (Scientific Procedures) Act 1986

This Act provides a system of controls over the use of living animals for experimental and other scientific research.

Medicines Act 1968

This is a licensing system for the manufacture, development, sale and supply of medicines, including those pesticides sold as animal medicines.

Poisons Act 1972

This Act controls the distribution of those pesticides scheduled as poisons.

Highly Flammable Liquids and Liquified Gases Regulations 1972

These Regulations lay down requirements on the marking of containers and storage accommodation for highly flammable liquids, including some pesticides.

Air Navigation Order 1974 and Rules of the Air and Air Traffic Control Regulations 1974

This controls the aerial application of pesticides. The Civil Aviation Authority document *The Aerial Application Permission –*

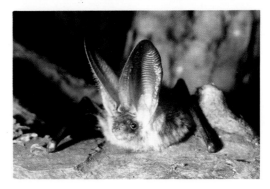

Bats are afforded special protection under the Wildlife and Countryside Act 1981 due to fears of their extinction.

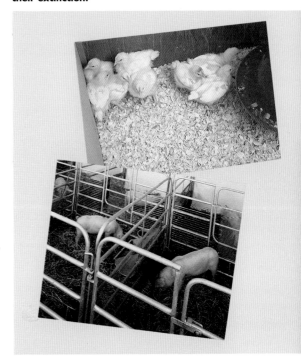

The Animals (Scientific Procedures) Act 1986 provides control over the use of living animals for research.

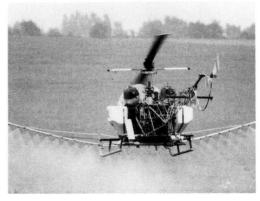

Aerial application of pesticides.

Requirements and Information contains a list of pesticides permitted for aerial spraying.

EUROPEAN COMMUNITY

European law is having an increasing impact on the national legislation and regulatory frameworks of the 12 Member States. The completion of the Single European Market in 1992, based on the Single European Act 1987, is likely to accelerate this process further. The central aim of the European Community (EC) is the creation of the free market for the movement of goods and services, persons and capital between Member States. Health, safety and environmental laws cannot be used as a barrier to free trade within the EC.

As a result, there is a potential source of conflict between health, safety and environmental requirements and those of free trade. The harmonisation of health, safety and environmental standards could mean, in practice, the lowest standards of the most poorly regulated member state being adopted as the norm. The EC has now taken over in large part from the Organisation for Economic Cooperation and Development (OECD) as the forum where the pesticide-exporting countries debate how much responsibility and regulation they are willing to assume for the international pesticide trade. EC countries account for 60% of world pesticide exports and so have a considerable influence. To date the EC has not enacted any form of export control, although it is to consider a mild form of Prior Informed Choice (PIC) in 1990. This would, in effect, leave the importing country with the option of requesting, or not requesting, information on a shipment of chemical about to be sent to it. If information was not requested, the chemical would still be sent.

The EC's own legislation on pesticides and related chemicals is based on a series of Directives, some of which have been translated into national legislation in the member states.

The directives can be divided into three broad subject areas:

1 Registration and approval.
2 Use.
3 Residues.

Registration

The first attempt at EC harmonization of pesticide approvals and testing took place in 1976 when a 'tandem' directive was issued, aiming to establish one list of approved products and another list containing prohibited substances. In the event, only the half of the Directive containing the list of banned substances was agreed. This Directive, known as the EC Plant Protection Prohibitions Directive 79/117/EEC, will be replaced by a Directive adopted in 1989.

The new EC Directive, Concerning the placing of EC-accepted (authorized) Plant Protection Products on the market, COM(89) 34 final, is due to come into effect in 1990. This new Directive provides for a base list of acceptable substances used as active ingredients in pesticides. It lays on Member States the duty of agreeing commonly accepted standards and protocols for testing pesticides, and sharing information. A procedure is set out for applicants to add new ingredients to the list of acceptable substances, and for reviewing all such substances within 10 years of the implementation of the Directive. Potentially, this could ensure uniform standards of testing, information exchange, pesticides registration requirements, and labelling. It could do away with the need to replicate toxicity testing, and so avoid the use of further laboratory test animals.

The essential proposals are that:

1 The EC will establish a positive list of pesticide active ingredients – used only for plant protection – which will be tested and authorized/approved to EC safety and efficacy standards.

2 Vetting of toxicological data and registration of pesticide active ingredients can be done by any of the national pesticide registration authorities, which will remain in existence.

3 Older pesticide active ingredients will be reviewed for safety over a 10-year period. They can only be placed on the positive, authorized list if they meet modern safety testing standards.

4 Sale of the 420 active ingredients, and products made from them, currently available in EC countries will still be allowed during this 10-year review period.

5 There will be a 'mutual acceptance' of authorized plant protection products in trade between member states.

6 Member states will not be able to refuse the import or use of authorised pesticide products on health and safety grounds. The only criterion for refusing to accept an authorised pesticide product is on special grounds of agricultural or climatic conditions.

7 An EC Standing Committee on Plant Protection will monitor the registration and acceptance of pesticide active ingredients and products in EC countries.

8 There will be a 10-year period of protection for manufacturers' safety data for new active ingredients, and a 5 year period for review information.

9 There is controversy between EC countries over the confidentiality of safety data. Some countries want full public access to basic toxicological and review data, while other governments and sections of the pesticide industry are arguing for strict confidentiality and safeguards.

10 Genetically-engineered micro-organisms used as pesticides are excluded, as these are covered in a separate EC Biotechnology Directive. Wood preservatives and industrial pesticides are excluded, along with veterinary pesticides.

Use

There have been no specific EC directives on pesticide use. However, the Control of Substances Hazardous to Health Regulations (COSHH) 1988 cover occupational pesticide manufacture, formulation and use in Great Britain; this legislation originated from an EC Directive.

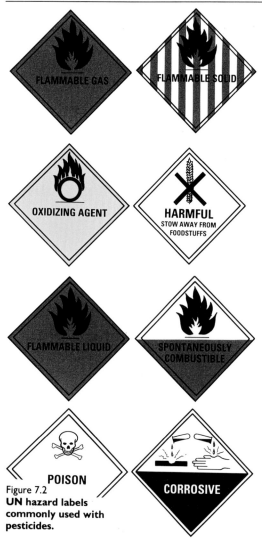

Figure 7.2
UN hazard labels commonly used with pesticides.

Residues

The EC has introduced a Framework Directive which aims to establish a set of mandatory Maximum Residue Levels (MRLs) for fruit and vegetables and certain other crops such as oilseeds and hops. It will make it easier to prescribe and alter maximum residue levels in food. Two earlier Directives which already set mandatory MRLs for animal products and cereals (incorporated into UK standards) will be reviewed as part of this process.

A priority list would be established for crops and pesticide active ingredients where there is currently no MRL. The UK Government has proposed the pesticide active ingredients maleic hydrazide and pirimiphos methyl as its top priorities for inclusion in the EC list. Existing MRLs for specific pesticides would be systematically reviewed to see whether the levels should be altered.

The full title of the Directive is: 4092/1/89 COM(88) 798, EC Proposal for the Council Regulation on the fixing of maximum levels for pesticide residues in and on certain products of plant origin, including fruit and vegetables, and amending Directive 76/895/EC as regards procedural rules.

Freedom of Information

A proposal has also been published by the Commission for a Directive on the freedom of access to information on the environment. This will enable individuals to obtain information about the environment held by public authorities, subject to safeguards in respect of trade and industrial confidentiality. It will also require governments to publish at least every 3 years from 1 January 1992 a report on the state of the environment containing a general analysis of the national situation, the state of water, air, soil, flora, fauna, and natural sites, and a description of the principal measures taken, or planned to preserve, protect, and improve the quality of the environment and to repair any damage caused.

WORLD HEALTH ORGANISATION

Within its mandate to co-operate with Member States on protection of health and prevention of health risks, the World Health Organisation (WHO) carries out a wide range of work under the heading of environment and health[284]. Safety assessment of pesticides carried out by WHO encompasses three main areas: hazard analysis and risk assessment (through the International Programme on Chemical Safety); hazard classification (Figure 7.2); and safety evaluation of pesticides in food. The work on pesticide residues began in 1961, when WHO held a joint meeting with the UN Food and Agricultural Organisation (FAO) on the use of pesticides in agriculture. Joint meetings have been held regularly since then, with reports published for most years since 1965. During the meetings, the FAO working party reviews data on selected pesticides and their residues, proposes pesticide residue limits, and recommends methods of analysis, while the WHO expert committee reviews toxicological data and establishes, wherever possible, acceptable daily intake levels (ADIs) and maximum residue levels

(MRLs). Although WHO has no legal authority over Member States, this yearly examination of data focuses international attention on the possible toxicological effects of pesticide residues, and has considerable moral authority.

New WHO *Guidelines for Predicting Dietary Intake of Pesticide Residues* were published in 1989[285]. Responsibility for establishing MRLs for pesticides in food falls on the Codex Committee on Pesticide Residues (CCPR), a subsidiary of the Codex Alimentarius Commission. The primary aim of the CCPR is to develop Codex Maximum Residue Limits (MRLs) as worldwide standards, in order to facilitate international trade while protecting the health of the consumer. WHO *Guidelines for Drinking Water Quality* were issued in 1984, based on toxicological data available up to 1981. Since that time new data have become available, but it has been concluded that the general philosophy of the 1984 guidelines remains valid, pending the publication of a revised edition.

FREEDOM OF INFORMATION

In the USA and other countries, including Australia, the existence of a Freedom of Information Act guarantees greater openness. Armed with this information, American pressure groups are ready to go to law. They can afford it because, compared with British campaigning organizations, they are rich. The Natural Resources Defense Council, which drew public attention to Alar[269], has revenues of $11 million a year. The American legal system also makes it easier for the 'little guy' to take on big business. A lawyer can be engaged on a no-win, no-charge contingency fee system, enabling individuals and groups to undertake litigation without the financial risks experienced in the UK.

US pesticide legislation provides for a very considerable degree of disclosure of pesticide safety data. Under the Federal Insecticide, Fungicide and Rodenticide Act (FIFRA), health and safety and environmental data submitted by manufacturers to the Environmental Protection Agency (EPA) is available to the public in full. However, the data are not disclosed to representatives of foreign or multinational pesticide companies, who might profit from it overseas. Those who receive the information are not allowed to publish it in full, but may summarize it or publish critiques. It is not just manufacturers' safety data that is now publicly available in the United States. In 1985 the EPA issued new rules to allow minutes of meetings between the EPA and outside parties, as well as correspondence, to be made available to the public[2].

Such information is available not only within the USA, but also to those requesting it from overseas (other than those with commercial interests). Indeed, Friends of the Earth was the first overseas enquirer to obtain full data on a pesticide (Monsanto's Roundup) from the EPA. It is ironic that British citizens can obtain information about the hazards they face at home from Washington DC, but access to information in the UK is considerably less well developed, despite some promising early signs. In 1984 the Tenth Report of the Royal Commission on Environmental Pollution[248] declared that there should be a 'presump-

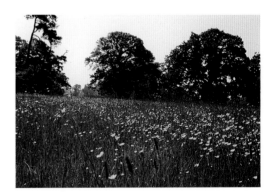

The public should have greater freedom of access to information on the state of the environment.

tion in favour of unrestricted access for the public to information which the pollution control authorities obtain by virtue of their statutory powers'. The Government accepted this guiding principle in consultation documents on implementing the Food and Environment Protection Act, and an inter-departmental working party recommended 'a significant shift in the direction of greater openness, fully in line with the Royal Commission's guiding principle'[286].

The agrochemical industry in the UK states that access to pesticide information in the UK is in fact more fully developed than the public seems to believe, and where data are not available there are good commercial reasons for this to be so. The *Pesticides Manual* published by the British Crop Protection Council and the *Agrochemical Handbook* published by the Royal Society of Chemistry are both easily available through libraries. Although in condensed form, toxicological properties are summarised in these volumes. Much more extensive information on toxicological and environmental factors may be found in the Reports and Evaluations of the Joint Meeting on Pesticide Residues of FAO/WHO. These reports and evaluations are obtainable from HMSO. In addition, detailed information is contained in *Environmental Health Criteria* published by WHO, Geneva. Under the provisions of the Control of Pesticide Regulations enquirers can receive from MAFF copies of the so-called 'Evaluation' document. This document comprises a detailed and comprehensive summary of all the regulatory data that have formed the basis of an approval granted under the Regulations. For reasons of confidentiality these documents cannot be used by third parties if they would be accessible to competitors in the UK and overseas.

In order to develop a new pesticide, research work of considerable complexity, novelty and extent is undertaken. With an investment in the order of millions of pounds in research and development, companies are understandably reluctant to allow potential competitors to have access to these data. This is the reason for the checks that exist, allowing access to regulatory data only to those who can satisfy appropriate criteria. Even in the USA it is not possible simply to walk into a government office and demand access to data under the Freedom of Information Act. Third parties have to sign an affidavit confirming reasons for requiring access to the data and affirming that it will not be used for any commercial purposes.

There is a strong case for public access to the safety test data submitted to Departments by manufacturers in connection with applications for pesticide approvals. Such access is needed so that there can be fully informed public discussion of the risks of pesticides and the adequacy of controls; so that those who have experienced or observed unexplained ill-effects can assess the likelihood that these result from pesticide exposure; and so that pesticide users can make informed choices from among the pesticides available to them[2]. To achieve these aims evaluations need to be made available for all pesticides currently in use. In fact, MAFF only releases information on pesticides as they are approved or reviewed. At present, some 3000 pesticide products, involving 400 active ingredients, are cleared for use. Information on their safety will only be released when they are reviewed in the future, and the pace at which reviews are being completed is painfully slow. In July 1989 the Department of Environment announced the establishment of an official Bureau of Environmental Information, similar to the Office of Population Censuses and Surveys, with the role of disseminating already published environmental statistics.

ENFORCEMENT AGENCIES

Health and Safety Executive

The Health and Safety Executive (HSE) is responsible for the promotion of health and safety in the workplace and for eliminating the risks to the public from work activities. In turn, responsibility for enforcement is shared between the various Inspectorates which make up the HSE. Those relevant to pesticides are:

1 *HSE Agricultural Inspectorate* – which enforces standards on pesticide storage and use on farms, in horticulture and forestry. Inspectors also deal with public complaints over spraying incidents – including aerial spraying – where there is alleged to have been a risk to human health.

2 *HSE Factory Inspectorate* – which enforces health and safety in pesticide manufacture and formulation industries. Also covered by the Factory Inspectorate is the use of pesticides in manufactured products, such as textiles and marine paints. Under the new pesticide laws, inspectors have additional powers to control the use by local authorities, public utilities, commercial pest control firms, and food storage facilities. They also deal with risks to the public from pesticide use in *parks and public places*.

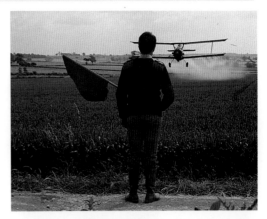

Public complaints regarding aerial crop spraying are dealt with by the Health and Safety Executive Agricultural Inspectorate.

Local authorities

Local authorities have new powers to control pesticide advertising, sale and use in domestic properties. They are also responsible for incidents arising from their storage, sale or use in offices, shops and commercial premises, including warehouses. More than one department could be involved – for example the Environmental Health Department and the Trading Standards Department.

Ministry of Agriculture Fisheries and Food (MAFF)

The Ministry of Agriculture, Fisheries and Food (MAFF) including its Agricultural Development and Advisory Service (ADAS), has responsibility for investigating incidents involving damage to domestic property, gardens or crops from spraying activities, as well as allegations that domestic animals or wildlife have been affected by pesticides. MAFF also has the power to seize or dispose of consignments of food shown to contain pesticide residues above the MRL.[287]

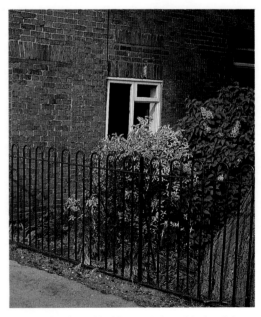

Investigation of incidents, such as this, involving damage to gardens by pesticides is the responsibility of the Agricultural Development and Advisory Service.

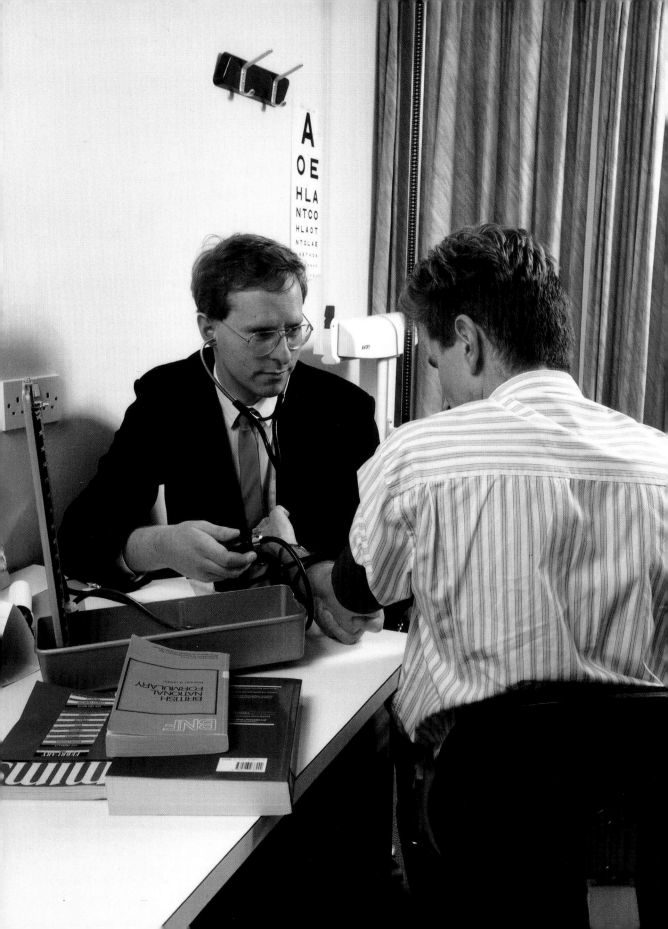

8 EDUCATION AND TRAINING

EDUCATING THE DOCTORS

The training of medical undergraduates in at least the basic principles of toxicology, as well as in the science and law relevant to pesticides, and in occupational and environmental health, is given a low priority. The General Medical Council booklet *Recommendations on Basic Medical Education* does not even mention toxicology, although aspects of the subject are covered in the recommendations on forensic pathology, legal medicine and pharmacology. At the present time no consultant physician is employed on a full-time NHS contract in clinical toxicology in the UK. Only about 12 are employed with part-time contracted commitments to this discipline. This provides a poor basis for training.

In 1988 Professor A. D. Dayan of the Department of Toxicology at St Bartholomew's Hospital sent a questionnaire to the Deans of undergraduate medical schools in Britain to ascertain the place of toxicology in the curriculum. All 24 medical schools replied to the questionnaire. Toxicology was defined for them as 'the study of the harmful effects on man of exposure to chemicals as medicines, at work, at home, in food, and in the environment.' To the question 'Do your undergraduates receive formal teaching about toxicology?' 22 replied 'Yes' and two 'No'. The number of hours given to teaching toxicology in complete medical courses in the 22 schools ranged from 12 hours at best, down to a single hour.

The teaching of toxicology and medicines was covered in all pharmacology courses, the amount of time allocated again varying from 12 hours to 1 hour. Toxicology and industry was covered in eight courses (occupational medicine/health four; community medicine four) with time allocated ranging from 1 to 10 hours. Consumer products were covered in five courses (pharmacology, community health, occupational medicine, medicine and forensic medicine) and were allocated as little as 15 minutes, at best 2 hours. Eight courses included attention given to foodstuffs (pharmacology three, clinical pharmacology, community medicine, forensic medicine, metabolic medicine). One course involved a visit to a food factory. The amount of time varied from a brief mention to 3 hours. The environment was covered in 11 courses (community medicine seven, pharmacology, two; biochemistry, one; chemical pathology, one). Here the time varied from 15 minutes to 4 hours[288].

The numbers in the survey were small and the questions sometimes misunderstood (Professor Dayan remains puzzled by a discounted response claiming 20 hours a year instruction on food toxicology in a psychiatry department). There is, however, a fairly consistent pattern of minimal attention to toxicology in general, and little if any formal coverage of it outside the area of pharmaceuticals. A teaching time of less than ten hours in an entire undergraduate course cannot equip a medical student to practise in this chemical age. Every year, the average healthy UK citizen feels ill enough to take at least three prescriptions and five proprietary medicines, each consisting of an active ingredient and several excipients (Figure 8.1); eats about 800 kg food (containing thousands of natural and synthetic substances); drinks at least 800 litres of water with traces of several hundred substances; breathes 7000 m³ air comprising two principal and eight minor gases and many contaminants; and has at least 15 chemical preparations at home for cleaning and so on. About 60 000 different materials may be used in industry, including up to 4000 handled in large amounts.

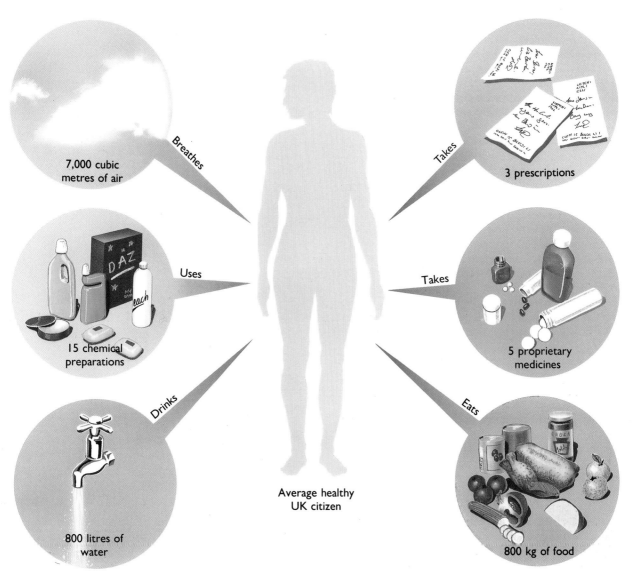

7,000 cubic metres of air

Breathes

Takes

3 prescriptions

Uses

Takes

15 chemical preparations

5 proprietary medicines

Drinks

Eats

800 litres of water

Average healthy UK citizen

800 kg of food

Figure 8.1
The average healthy UK citizen will receive a high chemical body load during any given year and doctors need to be aware of the possibility of disease resulting from exposure to these substances.

A more specific questionnaire survey[289] was undertaken in 26 medical schools in Great Britain in 1989 regarding medical teaching relative to the use of pesticides, and the possible effects on public health of exposure. Responses of some kind were received from 18 out of 26 schools (69%), and in 39.6% of cases questionnaire sections were returned.

All respondents were asked to answer attitudinal questions. A striking finding was how non-uniform is the concept of 'pesticide' among medical teachers (see Figure 8.2). Answers indicated some concerns that pesticide residues in food and water may be causing low-grade illness, and there was a diversity of views regarding the inadequacy of UK pesticide legislation. Pesticides in food ranked fourth, after atmospheric and drinking water pollution and infected food, as a public health issue. Food additives ranked fifth. There was a moderate level of agreement that we should be working towards an ecological/biological method of controlling pests and diseases, and some agreement that there is no fundamental distinction between natural and synthetic chemicals.

Some schools offered instruction in the effects of environmental pollution and nutrition on health. Most schools taught the basic scientific principles necessary to appreciate the factors determining the effects of low level exposures either in biochemistry or pharmacology. In biochemistry, an average of 5.7 hours of instruction was given on the metabolism and detoxification of compounds absorbed into the body. Only two out of ten schools responding undertook any teaching in the role of pesticides in the control of vector-borne diseases or food spoilage and contamination, or on the regulations controlling their marketing and use. In internal and family medicine courses all respondents agreed that students were, and should be, expected to consider environmental factors in patient assessment. Some schools dealt with the environmental topics in postgraduate courses or meetings.

Clearly, there is an awareness of the importance of environmental issues in medicine and medical education, but teaching on these aspects has not achieved an agreed place in the curriculum. Indeed, there are indications of confusion over the whole issue of 'micropollution' and whether it should have a place in the curriculum. Pesticides are not regarded as micropollutants which require priority attention in the UK.

Not all doctors need to be expert toxicologists, but all doctors need to be aware of the possibility of disease resulting from toxic substances, and to have more training and practical experience in the differential diagnosis and treatment of chemically induced diseases. In particular, there should be greater awareness of the DHSS booklet *Pesticide Poisoning: Notes for the Guidance of Medical Practitioners*[111]. The first edition was distributed free of charge to every doctor in the NHS and a new edition is in preparation.

TRAINING THE WORKERS

One of the most important aspects of improving pesticides safety is in the proper training of all those handling the chemicals. The COSHH Regulations 1988 state that:

> 'An employer who undertakes work which may expose any of his employees to substances hazardous to health shall provide that employee with such information, instruction and training as is suitable and sufficient for him to know –
> a) the risks to health created by such exposure; and
> b) the precautions which shall be taken.'

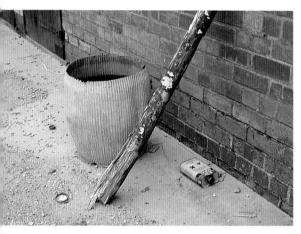

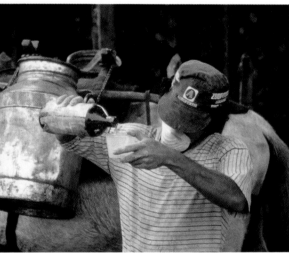

One of the most important aspects of pesticide safety is the proper training of all those handling the chemicals.

In the *Code of Practice for the Safe Use of Pesticides on Farms and Holdings in Great Britain* ('Green Code')[282] produced by MAFF and the Health and Safety Commission, the onus is on employers to provide adequate training in the safe handling of chemical pesticides. The Code identifies the following five areas in which workers require instruction and training: the relevant legislation; the hazards and risks posed by different pesticides; safe working practices to minimise these hazards; emergency action; and health surveillance and record keeping.

Training in Legislation

Users, which includes both employers and operators, should be familiar with those aspects of the Regulations made under Part III of the Food and Environment Protection Act for controlling the use of pesticides; COSHH, and other legislation that applies to the storage, transport, handling, use and disposal of pesticides. In addition, they should be aware that detailed requirements applying to use may be changed from time to time by variations in the conditions attached to product approvals or by changes in exposure limits.

Training in the Hazards and Risk of Pesticides

Users should be familiar with:

1 The product to be used and especially its potential hazards to human beings, animals, crops, other plants, beneficial insects, other wildlife, and the environment generally.
2 The nature and degree of the risks to health arising from exposure to pesticides, including any factors such as smoking which may influence those risks.

Training in Safe Working Practices

Users should be aware of and where necessary trained in:

1 The correct procedures for storing, handling and mixing pesticides, and the disposal of empty containers, other contaminated materials and surplus pesticides, whether in concentrate or dilute form.
2 The procedures for preparing application equipment for work, including its calibration, and for its operation without risk to the operator, other people, animals, beneficial insects, or the environment.
3 The control measures adopted to protect the operator, the reasons for them and how to use them properly.
4 The reasons for personal protective equipment (PPE), including clothing, its selection, and the jobs where it is necessary.
5 The safety procedures to be followed before, during and after application, recognizing the conditions where pesticide use could pose a risk to people, animals, beneficial insects, plants and the environment including water, and the need to avoid use in such circumstances.
6 The correct procedure for cleaning and storing clothing or equipment which may be contaminated.
7 The procedures for monitoring, including access to results and whether the exposure limit has been exceeded.

Training in Emergency Action

Users should be trained in:

1 The emergency action necessary in the event of a spillage of concentrated or dilute pesticide.
2 The emergency action necessary to decontaminate people, the known signs and symptoms of pesticide poisoning and the action to be taken, including where to obtain medical advice in the event of accidental poisoning.

Training in Health Surveillance and Record Keeping

Users should be aware of and receive training in:

1 The role of health surveillance, the need to undertake health surveillance, and the provision of access, subject to the right of confidentiality of personal health information, to the records and results of health surveillance.
2 Completing records to meet statutory obligation. The information should also be made available to employees' representatives in accordance with the Safety Representatives and Safety Committees Regulations 1977, where applicable.

Suitable training courses are provided by the Agricultural Training Board, agricultural colleges, and other bodies. Employers may provide their own training; this should be to an equivalent standard and should be adequately recorded.

The importance of training cannot be overstated, with regards to pesticide safety. The majority of accidents involving pesticides at work have occurred as a result of inadequate training and supervision. This is the message that is stated clearly in the Code of Practice on Pesticides:

'Everyone involved in the use of pesticides . . . must have adequate instruction and guidance in the safe, efficient and humane use of pesticides and be competent for the tasks they are called upon to perform.'

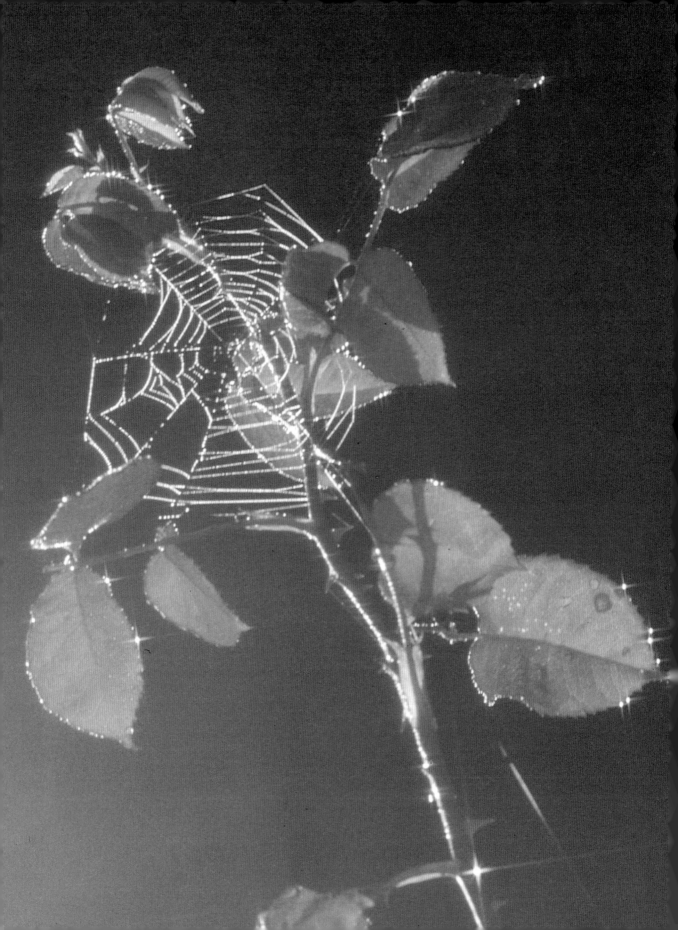

9 ALTERNATIVES TO CONVENTIONAL PESTICIDES FOR PEST CONTROL

A prolonged chemical warfare exists between insects and plants, and an equivalent coevolution of plant defences and of means of detoxifying them. Indeed, some insects have evolved methods of dealing with plant toxins which make them resistant to chemical control. More than 500 insect pests are now at least partially resistant to chemical control[290] and, in the search for new solutions, attention is increasingly focusing on non-chemical methods of plant protection: preventative methods, organic farming, biological control, and genetic engineering (a form of chemical control using the plant's own biochemistry). The combination of these 'alternative methods' with the best of modern chemical techniques is often called 'integrated pest management'. Many of the agrochemical companies are now investing in research and development of biological and microbial pesticides, and in biotechnology. However, according to industry estimates these approaches are unlikely to account for more than 5% of the total crop protection market by the turn of the century[64]. Most pest control will be chemically based for the forseeable future, with an emphasis on product substitution of highly active and specific pesticides for older chemical formulations.

INTEGRATED PEST MANAGEMENT

Pragmatic and effective approaches to plant protection are being achieved under the broad heading of 'integrated pest management' (IPM). IPM takes traditional cultural methods, such as crop rotation, fallowing, manual weeding, intercropping and the encouragement of natural predators, and combines them with (and modifies them by) modern chemical techniques. Briefly, IPM 'embraces any combination of artificial and natural controls to produce the greatest advantage'[291].

Many good examples of IPM are older than the phrase (first used in 1959)[292]. In Britain, sugar beet is protected by a combination of methods. Seed beet is planted far away from beet used for sugar to prevent transfer of aphids between the crops. Routine field surveys are carried out by trained workers,

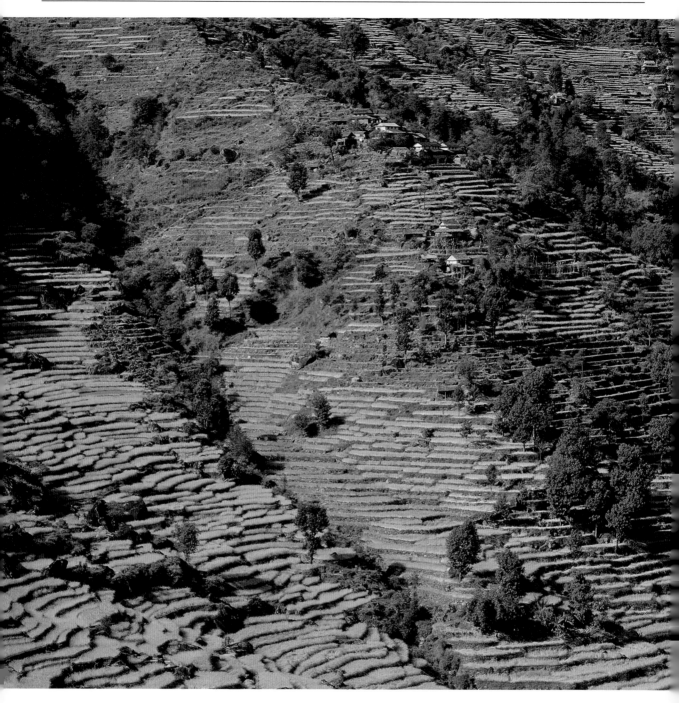

Fish and ducks used in paddy fields have proven a more effective, less costly and less harmful method of pest control.

and if more than one aphid is found per four plants then a systemic insecticide is applied. The British Sugar Corporation also requires all planting to be done on land on which no beet or brassica has been grown in the previous 2 years[293].

There are many examples of effective IPM in the developing world. Chinese agriculture has used IPM based on careful studies of breeding insects, exclusion tactics and biological controls, combined with the use of a small number of chemical pesticides. Fish and ducks are used to control pests in paddy fields. China grows 39% of the world's rice, yet in 1980 was

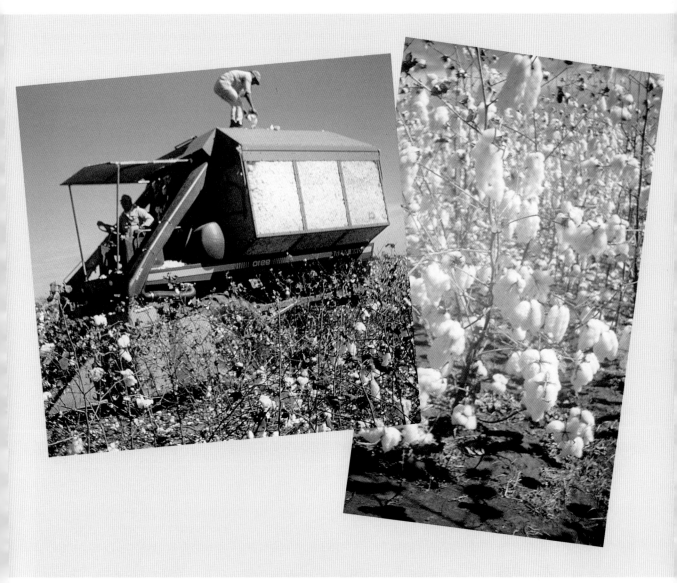

Integrated pest management schemes have been effectively introduced in Nicaragua to protect the cotton crop.

reported as relying on only seven organophosphorus insecticides[294]. In Cuba the entire sweet potato acreage is under biological control. For peppers and sweet corn, alternate planting dates reduced pesticide applications from 28 to 12 in 1983. The sugar borer has been controlled by parasites since 1977. The citrus fruit blackfly is also controlled biologically, allowing the number of fungicide applications to be reduced from 15 to one or two a year[295]. Since the 1970s effective IPM schemes have been introduced in Nicaragua. The cotton crop is protected by closer supervision and monitoring, together with physical trapping of boll weevils. Chemical pesticides are used in conjunction with these techniques, although expenditure on these has dropped by 50% since the 1970s[296].

In the Canete Valley in Peru, entomologists have devised methods to reduce the amount spent on pesticides to 3–5% of the total production costs of the cotton crop. Regular checks of the fields are made to monitor the levels of pests and beneficial insects. Quarantine posts prevent the spread of diseased plant material, and there are strict regulations to control the time of planting and harvest. Farmers have cut their use of insecticides down to one or two sprays per season. After two seasons yields of cotton were back to the levels expected during the period of heavy chemical use in the 1950s, when farmers were spending about 30% of their production costs on organochlorine insecticides. The Canete experience has been the most serious trial of IPM in the world and its success has made it the textbook example of IPM for entomologists.

Effective integrated pest management strategies like these can provide an alternative to relying solely on chemical pesticide usage[297]. In the developed world the demand for inexpensive food, with a very high standard of freedom from pest damage, is such that approaches like biological control alone are unlikely to make a significant impact. A combination of the best of the 'chemical' and 'organic' worlds in an IPM approach may be the way forward.

PREVENTATIVE METHODS

In agriculture, as in health care, prevention is the best form of cure. Preventative methods of pest control have a long history.

Intercropping and diversity

Traditional farming systems are characterized by a diversified agricultural environment. In the fields a wide variety of crops (in terms of space and time) may be grown. Wild plants also add

Black grass control in field beans.

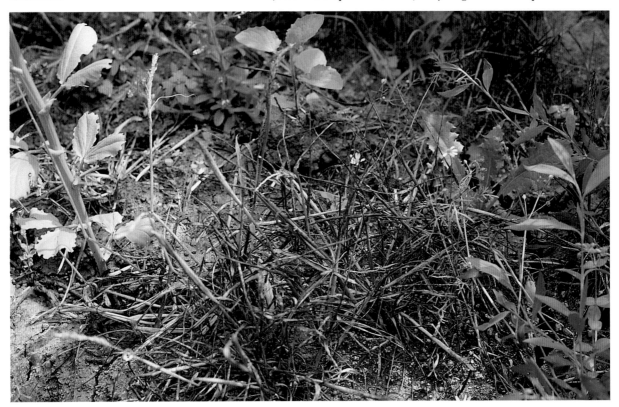

to this diversity. There are several reasons why intercropping systems are a good method of preventative crop protection[298]. A variety of small niches are created so that they attract the natural enemies of crop pests. Intercropping also produces a variety of visual and chemical stimuli which confuses pests which are unable to recognize their host plants. Care must be taken, however, with combinations of plants. Unsuitable intercropping can actually increase pest damage. In Costa Rica research into good combinations of plants has gone on for many years, and crop associations such as maize with beans, and cassava with sweet potato have proved to be particularly appropriate. In West Africa intercropping of maize and cowpeas has led to a significant reduction in pest damage[298]. In the UK, research by the Henry Doubleday Research Association into 'companion planting' has proved inconclusive. One of the few companionships that has been fully researched is onions intercropped with carrots. The onions do seem to protect the carrots from carrot-fly, but only with careful attention to spacing and timing. There must be two rows of onions each side of the carrots and the effect only lasts as long as the onions are growing leaves.

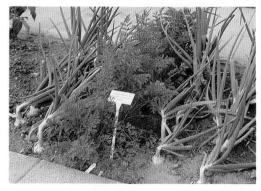

Onions may be intercropped with carrots to afford protection from carrot fly.

Cultivation practices

Other suitable cropping techniques can assist pest control[299].

Crop rotation and fallowing interrupts the lifecycle of pests and the continuity of pest population growth. It is the young of many pests rather than the adults that cause the damage, and in addition the appearance of pests and diseases are often associated with a particular stage of development in the host plant.

Timely sowing or planting reduces the possibility of pest reproduction coinciding with this stage of development in the plant. For example, the pea moth only lays eggs on pea flowers. By sowing early or late, the peas are not flowering from mid-June to mid-July when the moths are laying. Infected plant material left lying around can pass on pests and diseases to future crops. Field hygiene is basic good husbandry.

Choice of resistant varieties, where available, is also a sensible practice, as is the selection of appropriate varieties for the local conditions.

Physical methods

The earliest crop protection methods were of a physical kind. At the simplest level there was hand weeding and picking off insect pests by hand. Although in developed countries hand weeding would be unrealistic on a commercial scale, with prohibitively high labour costs, in Third World countries this is still an important approach and can be more cost effective than the application of pesticides. In mango plantations in Thailand, workers catch the fruit piercing moth in nets. This provides some local people with a living and overall costs of pest control have been calculated as approximately 5% of the cost of applying chemical pesticides[300]. Another technique, popular with organic gardeners, is the variety of ingenious barriers and traps (such as netting to keep out birds, squares of carpet around the base of brassica plants to give protection from

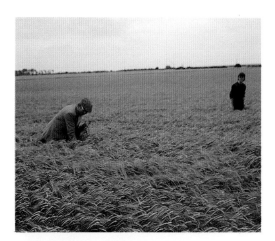

Hand weeding or 'Rouging' is backbreaking, monotonous and exhausting work.

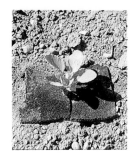

Squares of carpet provide protection from cabbage root fly.

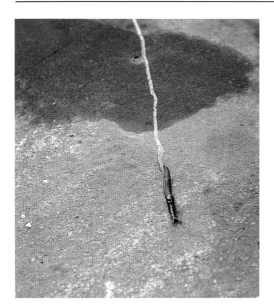

Traps filled with beer are reported to be an effective method of controlling slug damage.

cabbage root fly, and barriers of egg shell or soot, together with traps filled with beer for slugs).

The Boxworth Project

An investigation of the ecological and economic outcomes of different pesticide regimes in cereal farming was started in 1981 by the Agricultural Development and Advisory Service (ADAS) in collaboration with universities and an AFRC research institute at MAFF's Boxworth Experimental Husbandry Farm in Cambridgeshire. After monitoring the plant and animal populations for two years under the prevailing normal farm pesticide regimes, to provide a baseline for the subsequent treatments, the farm was divided into 3 large blocks. In years three to seven, one block received a high input 'Full Insurance' pesticide regime (with spraying to a preplanned schedule), another received a 'Supervised' control regime under which pesticides were only applied if thresholds for serious economic damage by pests were reached, and the third block, an 'Integrated' regime was similar to the 'supervised' one but husbandry operations and varieties were changed to further reduce the need for pesticides. Birds, small mammals, invertebrates and hedgerow plants as well as levels of particular pests, weeds and diseases were monitored throughout the study[301].

One important effect of the 'Full Insurance' high pesticide regime, compared with the more 'environmentally friendly', supervised and integrated regimes, was a decline in many beneficial predatory invertebrates in the fields heavily treated with pesticides. Although total insect herbivores also declined in this plot, there were signs that in later years the reduction in natural predators would result in higher and more frequent outbreaks of aphids and certain other pests.

There was some criticism of the project shown by the House of Lords Science and Technology Committee in 1984, who questioned the experiment design[302].

The Government replied to the Committee in 1985.[303] The project 'was not designed to provide definitive answers to all the questions raised in this area . . . as a test bed, it should identify those parts of the cereal ecosystem requiring further detailed study of pesticide effects'.

The economic results of the study were encouraging evidence for the potential of reduced and more rational use of pesticides. Wheat yields were greatest in the Full Insurance plot, but the additional costs of the spraying on this regime meant that an equal or slightly higher gross margin could be obtained instead in the Supervised regime. Both gave higher gross margins than the Integrated plot but this treatment differed in a variety of ways apart from pesticide regime, including wheat variety.

Although chosen on pragmatic ground, one important drawback of the simple three plot experimental design at Boxworth is that 'the lack of replication at a field scale limits the confidence with which results from Boxworth can be extrapolated to other conditions'. However, it should be particularly noted that some smaller, fully replicated trials at Boxworth gave very similar results and conclusions to the main study.

BIOLOGICAL CONTROL

Biological control makes use of natural predators to control the pest population. Definitions include Bull's 'classical biological control entails introducing an enemy of a pest for the purpose of controlling that pest'[45] and King and Coleman's 'biological control is the management of biological control agents (predators, parasites and microbial organisms) and their products to reduce pest population densities and their effects. This definition does not include genetic approaches, host plant resistance, or cultural control, nor does it include physical or chemical control except where these approaches supplement or affect natural enemies'[304].

The greatest successes in biological control have been achieved in relatively closed environments: oceanic islands with few species of plants and animals (even large islands like Australia and Hawaii), 'ecological islands' like California, shut off by deserts, mountains or seas; and on a domestic scale, within glasshouses[291]. An early example of successful biological control is the cottony cushion scale in California. This pest was accidentally introduced to California in 1868 on acacia plants from Australia. It spread to citrus trees so successfully that by 1886 citrus farmers faced ruin. An entomologist sent to Australia to discover why the scale gave no trouble there returned in 1889 with a consignment of ladybirds. These provided quite satisfactory control and there was no need for further effort or expenditure[305]. This spectacular demonstration of applied ecology established the practicality of biological pest control. A recent centennial review article has described it as 'unparalleled in the annals of entomology for its drama, human interest, political ramifications and continuing significance'[306]. About the same time the European gypsy moth was introduced into the Eastern USA and quickly established itself on forest trees. By 1923 some 75 million insects from 45 species had been introduced in an attempt to control the pest biologically, without success. It was not until DDT was sprayed from aircraft that the damage was checked. Since the banning of DDT the forest destruction has begun again. The introduction of natural predators without thorough prior investigation can sometimes produce a two-edged sword. In Queensland, Australia an attempt to control insect pests by introducing the cane toad resulted in the toads themselves becoming major pests.

Insect predators can also be used to control weeds. The best known case of biological control of weeds is the control of several species of prickly pear which, having originated in the USA, had spread over 40 million hectares of grazing land in Australia by 1925. Much of this land was unusable and in some places the cactus was impenetrable. Imported enemies of the prickly pear, amounting to half a million insects of about 50 species, helped little. Then, quite unexpectedly, an Argentinian cactus eating moth *(Cactoblastis cactorum)* destroyed the prickly pears so effectively that no other remedy was needed[291]. It should be borne in mind that the prickly pears were themselves organisms released carelessly into a new terrain, and there is a lesson to be learned here about the possible adverse consequences of importing alien species.

T. H. C. Taylor became well known for his successful

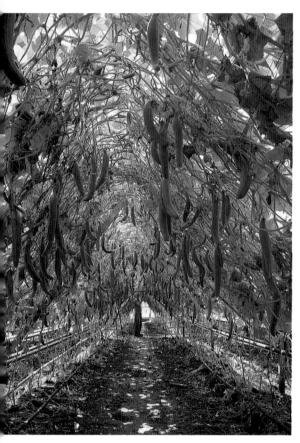

Biological control has been successfully used to protect greenhouse cucumbers and tomatoes.

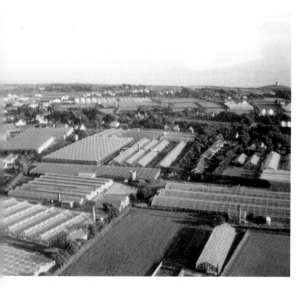

Biological controls are now being adopted by commercial glasshouse growers.

introductions of controlling insects into the island of Fiji in the 1930s. After many years of work on biological control he concluded that it was the best of all possible methods when it worked, but that it did not work often enough for it to have much future in continental areas[307]. There has, however, been a recent example of successful biological pest control in the African continent. Cassava is a staple crop for millions of people in Africa. It was afflicted with mealy bug and green mite that had been brought in from South America in the 1970s. After research, a parasitic wasp was found which preyed on the pests and saved the crop. Yields were restored and hardship to the population on a large scale was prevented[308]. There is a well-documented recent example of the introduction to Israel during 1976–87 of more than 200 shipments of beneficial insects for the biological control of soft-scale insects, armoured scale insects, whitefly, aphids, mealybugs and Mediterranean fruit fly. Of these, 60 species were successfully cultured in laboratories at the Israel Cohen Institute for Biological Control and, so far, six are well established and have effected successful biological control of *Saissetia oleae* and *Dialeurodes citri*[309].

Within the UK the outstanding success is the control system for mites and insects on greenhouse cucumbers and tomatoes. Two of the most troublesome pests affecting the commercial production of cucumbers and tomatoes are the glasshouse whitefly and the red spider mite. Not only do they cause an immense amount of damage but they have also proved intractable to effective chemical control. Fortunately there have been considerable successes with the introduction of predators. In the case of the red spider mite it is another predatory mite *(Phytoseilus persimilis)*, while whitefly is controlled by a tiny wasp called *Encarsia formosa*. These biological controls are now rapidly being taken up by commercial glasshouse and polytunnel growers. From being used hardly at all a decade ago, *Encarsia* is now used on over half the UK cucumber crop and 43% of tomatoes. The figures for the red spider predator are 63% and 14% respectively. Packs containing stocks of both predators, *Encarsia* and *Phytoseilus*, are now cheaply available, even for the amateur gardener, from suppliers such as the Henry Doubleday Research Association.

Biological pest control extends beyond the use of beneficial insects to include smaller organisms (fungi, bacteria, viruses) which may themselves act as parasites on insect pests. Attempts were made in Russia in 1879 to use a fungus *(Metarrhizium anisopliae)* against cockchafers; in Kansas from 1890 to use another fungus *(Beauveria bassiana)* against the chinch bug; and in Central America in 1910 to use a bacterium *(Coccobacillus acridiorum)* to control locusts. Today a bacterium *(Bacillus popilliae)* is used in the USA to control Japanese beetle on golf courses and lawns[291].

Many known viruses attack insects. The best known are the nuclear polyhedrosis viruses (NPV), but there are also the granulosis viruses (GV), and 136 other kinds. The NPV and GV are found only in insects and are unlikely to harm other organisms. Some of the others can cause serious diseases in sheep, fish, plants and fungi, while certain pox viruses which are effective against insects can also kill humans. For this reason it is only the NPV and GV classes that have been much tested against insects[310]. The most valuable introduction of a virus actually occurred accidentally. Insect parasites taken from Europe to Canada in an attempt to control European spruce sawfly were found to carry a virus which was in itself very effective in controlling the sawfly. It has now been introduced to other parts of the USA and Canada and is the main controlling agent. Another celebrated example of the use of viruses in pest control is the introduction of a viral disease, myxomatosis, from South America to control rabbits in Australia[291]. The decimation of the UK rabbit population by myxomatosis would of course be regarded by many as a heavy price to pay for effective biological pest control.

Viruses are most useful where some degree of damage can be tolerated and where the value of the crop is not great enough to bear the cost of chemical pesticides. On the whole, insect viruses seem to be fairly specific. This is advantageous in that their attack is confined to the target species, but disadvantageous in that cost of development and testing could seldom be recouped in controlling a single species. Today attention is focused on the highly specific Baculoviruses and *Bacillus thuringiensis*. Although discovered many years ago these organisms are increasingly integrated into biological pest control. Some experts have estimated that, on a worldwide scale, approximately 30% of all agricultural and woodland pests could be combated with the help of Baculoviruses[311]. In Brazil Baculovirus preparations are industrially manufactured for soya cultivation and are applied to over one million hectares. In the USA Sandoz now manufacture and distribute an NPV called Elcar, which has been approved for the control of bollworms in cotton cultivation. *Bacillus thuringiensis* preparations currently on the market are Thuricide HP (Sandoz), Dipel (Abbott) and Bactospeine (Biochem)[298].

SEMIOCHEMICALS

Another approach to controlling pests is to modify their behaviour by exploiting their natural chemical communication or feeding cues. Semiochemicals are non-toxic behaviour modifying chemicals such as sex pheromones, used by insect females to attract their mates, and antifeedants (compounds that interfere with feeding behaviour) which may be based on the compounds produced by plants.

Pheromones

Lepidopteran sex pheromones are perhaps the best known. In many moth species the females release pheromones (odours) and in response males fly up wind to find them. For some species these compounds have been identified and synthesized. Such pheromones have been used in four main ways: for monitoring populations, for disrupting mating, for mass trapping, and for 'lure and kill'[312,313].

Monitoring

Insect pheromones, placed in traps as bait, are used for the detection of pest insects and monitoring their numbers. As part of an integrated pest management system this information can be used to time the best application of conventional pesticides (thereby reducing use) or, if the pest is shown not to be present or at levels unlikely to cause economic damage, not used at all. For example, in the UK a practical pheromone monitoring system has been developed for the pea moth, *Cydia nigricana*[314].

Mating Disruption

If sufficient synthetic pheromone is released into the crop the male moths may find it difficult to find and fertilize females. This leads to a reduction of the damaging caterpillar stage, but without killing natural enemies (predators and parasitoids) in the crop, which are left able to control the remaining caterpillars and other pests. This has been used with success with the pink bollworm, *Pectinophora gossypiella*[311].

Mass Trapping

In this technique traps baited with pheromone are used to trap out the pest population, but despite many trials on both Lepidoptera and forest bark beetles success has been limited[312].

Lure and Kill

These techniques use pheromones to attract the pest to a limited area treated with insecticide. In this way the area treated is greatly reduced.

Alarm Pheromones

These compounds, produced by some insect species, stimulate escape and other defence behaviours. They have been used experimentally in two ways.[315] First, synthetic honey-bee alarm pheromone components have been used to protect bees from contact with pesticides by repelling them from newly sprayed crops, but with limited success. Second, and more successfully, aphid alarm pheromones have been added to contact insecticides resulting in an increase in mortality because the aphids' escape activity brought them into more contact with the insecticide treated leaves.

Antifeedants

Many plants have compounds that deter herbivorous insects and much effort is going into identifying the compounds and devising methods for using them in crop protection. For example, it has proved possible to protect barley from aphid-borne virus disease by spraying it with the antifeedant compounds such as polygodial which are produced by the plant water-pepper (*Polygonum hydropiper*)[315].

Currently semiochemicals appear to be most effective as part of integrated pest management programmes in which they can make significant reductions in conventional pesticide use. However, in some cases, such as the use of pheromones for mating disruption in the cotton pest Pectinophora, the pheromone treatments were as good as insecticides in controlling the pest and highly satisfactory yields were obtained[312] and thus here pheromones might even replace conventional pesticides.

BIOTECHNOLOGY AND GENETIC CONTROL

Genetic approaches to pest control involve altering the characteristics of an organism, through breeding or through more sophisticated genetic engineering. The main techniques are the breeding of resistant plants, and the genetic engineering of one generation of insect pest to reduce the population in the next.

Breeding resistant plants

For many years agriculturalists and scientists have sought to increase crop yields through plant breeding programmes. Increased yields can come from plants that stand up better to adverse weather conditions, respond better to fertilizers, or resist attack by pests and diseases. The best known breeding programmes for resistance are those in the USA where varieties of wheat have been produced which are able to resist attacks of black stem-rust. Unfortunately, the stem-rust produces its own new varieties which overcome the resistance bred into the wheat. Wheat breeders have to produce new varieties frequently to meet this recurring challenge[291].

Resistance to insect attack is much more difficult to achieve, but a variety of cotton plant has been developed which is resistant to attack by leafhoppers[316]. There has, however, been considerable interest in a novel pesticide developed by Monsanto in the USA (the engineered 'insecticidal plant'). Their starting point was the *Bacillus thuringiensis* (Bt) bacterium which has been used by agriculturalists for over 20 years to control gypsy moth and other caterpillars on plants such as cabbage, cotton, beans and potatoes. This form of biological control has no effect on animals and plants other than the target species at which it is directed. Furthermore, it does not persist in the environment. The disadvantage is that crops must be sprayed repeatedly to ensure their continued protection. What the researchers at Monsanto Agricultural Products have managed to do is to clone the gene responsible for the organism's toxicity and to transfer it to *Pseudomonas fluorescens*, a harmless bacterium which has the useful ability to colonize plant roots. Applied at the time of planting, the engineered organism can thus afford long-term protection against soil-borne pests. Further research is needed before we know more about whether there is a possibility of the gene being transferred to other plants or insects[317], or whether the target insect population will in time develop resistance to Bt[318].

A further possibility now being studied at several centres is to create plants with heightened tolerance to herbicides. Pesticides vary greatly in their effects on different species of plants. They can thus be employed as selective weed killers for purposes such as preventing broad-leaved plants growing on lawns. However, the crop must, of course, be resistant to the herbicide used to protect it, and such tolerance has been an important goal of both herbicide design and plant breeding. Several herbicides sprayed on corn in the American corn belt persist sufficiently to affect soybeans sowed the following year. This has stimulated efforts to breed soybeans with greater resistance to the particular herbicide. Conventional methods of doing this are limited

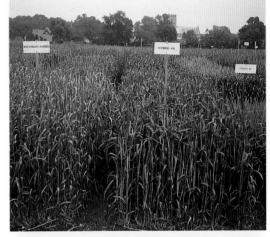

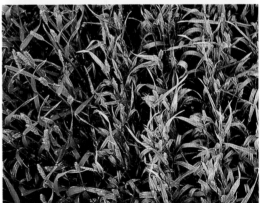

Genetic approaches to pest control includes the breeding of resistant plants.

but there have been successes in using DNA techniques, using genes from a far wider range of donors.

Genetic control of insect pest

These methods work by interfering genetically with one generation of insects to reduce the population in the next. The best known method is the release of great numbers of the pest species that have been sterilized by gamma rays or chemicals, so that they mate with no progeny and exhaust the reproductive capacity of their fertile wild mates. In the 1950s there was an extensive experiment using this technique to control screwworm attacking cattle in the Southern USA. This entailed rearing, sterilization by gamma ray and release from aircraft of 150 million flies per day at the height of the action. One hundred tonnes of horsemeat and 10 tonnes of dried blood were needed every week just to feed the flies. The dose of gamma rays had to be controlled with great care so as to sterilize the male flies without impairing their vigour in copulation.

Although the programme was very costly, not least because the flies kept migrating into Mexico, it was very effective for some years. In 1972, for unknown reasons, the control of screwworm broke down and something close to the original amount of damage was soon occurring annually[319]. The expense of using such large scale radiation techniques may be overcome by sterilization by feeding certain chemicals. Unfortunately, many of the available sterilizing chemicals act by producing mutations, which can occur in mammals, including human beings, as well as in insects. Some are also carcinogenic. They cannot consequently be used with bait or they might get into human food or be eaten by pets or wildlife[291].

The world's first commercial pesticide based on a live, genetically engineered organism is now on sale in New South Wales. The product, which protects stone fruits, nuts and roses from crown gall disease, is based on a benign strain of *Agrobacterium tumefaciens*. This produces an antibiotic which kills a pathogenic cousin of *A. tumefaciens*. Farmers normally poison it by gassing plants with ethylene bromide. Now they can control the *A. tumefaciens* which causes crown gall disease by soaking the roots of seedlings in a solution of the new product (NoGall) before planting. The department of agriculture in New South Wales cleared the product for sale without asking to examine toxicological or safety data from the manufacturers, Bio-Care Technology. The company is now confident of obtaining a licence to retail NoGall throughout Australia, and is also hoping for approval from the Environmental Protection Agency to sell the product in the USA.

Concern that genetically engineered organisms (GEOs) should be properly scrutinized for environmental and health effects before release prompted the publication in July 1989 of the Royal Commission on Environmental Pollution's thirteenth report, entitled *The Release of Genetically Engineered Organisms to the Environment*[320]. The report discusses the effects such a release might have on the environment, the procedures necessary to identify, assess and minimize any risks to the environment and human health, and the regulatory arrangements needed to ensure environmental protection. Recognizing that the environmental impact of released organisms may have undesirable as well as beneficial effects, the report stated that 'it would be prudent to begin with the assumption that an introduced gene could spread widely'. The Royal Commission did not feel that this indicated a moratorium on releases but instead considered it 'essential that the release of genetically engineered organisms (GEOs) is conducted from the outset under appropriate statutory control'.

The proposed framework for such a system of statutory control is a system of licences for release, or for product approval, to be granted by the Secretary of State for the Environment, in consultation with the Health and Safety Executive. Local committees based within the organization developing the GEO would screen proposals for release and refer well thought out proposals to a national committee of experts, the Release Committee. The Release Committee would have expert knowledge of genetic engineering techniques, microbiology, field ecology, and other relevant disciplines, and would be drawn from universities, government departments, industry, workers' representatives, and local authority environmental health officers. Proposals would be assessed by the Release Committee with regard to environmental protection and human health and safety, and recommendations made to Ministers. The Committee would advise on policy matters, develop codes of practice, review releases that had been licensed, and produce an annual report. A register would be compiled of all companies or organizations granted authority to release GEOs. These bodies would be obliged to satisfy criteria of training, safety, and the establishment of local committees. The government rejected the Royal Commission's call for the public to be notified of applications for GEO product approval.

The EC is presently considering three further directives relating to the safety aspects of biotechnology. There is a 'workplace directive' which seeks to protect workers from risks related to exposure to biological agents at work (Off. Jo. E.C. 1988 C 150/6). Two harmonization directives cover the use of GEOs in contained facilities (Official Journal of the European Communities 1988 C 198/9) and the deliberate release of GEOs to the environment (Official Journal of the European Communities 1988 C 198/19).

ORGANIC FARMING

What we describe as conventional agriculture is in fact of recent origin. With the appearance of cheap fertilizers at the end of the Second World War and cheap pesticides in the early 1950s, advanced countries quickly abandoned traditional or organic methods and became heavily dependent on both agrochemicals and labour-saving machinery. This was not because organic methods did not work but because they were not competitive enough. However, the modern concept of organic farming is not a return to some past golden age but rather a marriage of scientific advances with many traditional practices. The US Department of Agriculture regards organic farming as a system that avoids or excludes the use of synthetic fertilizers and pesticides, and relies upon practices such as crop rotation, the

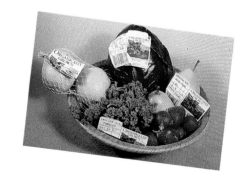

Organically grown produce is now available in most high street supermarkets.

use of animal and green manures, and some form of biological pest control.

Organic farmers have long claimed that they can achieve crop yields that are close to, or even equivalent to, those achieved in systems using agrochemicals. However, with virtually no research and development expenditure on organic farming systems since the Second World War this has been almost impossible to verify. Now a report from the US National Academy of Sciences, called *Alternative Agriculture*[321], has given support to the high productivity of organic farming. For the purposes of the report 'alternative agriculture' is defined as any system of food or fibre production that systematically pursues the following goals:

1 More thorough incorporation of natural processes such as nutrient cycles, nitrogen fixation, and pest–predator relationships into the agricultural production process.
2 Reduction in the use of off-farm inputs with the greatest potential to harm the environment or the health of farmers and consumers.
3 Greater productive use of the biological and genetic potential of plant and animal species.
4 Improvement of the match between cropping patterns and the productive potential and physical limitations of agricultural lands to ensure long-term sustainability of current production levels.
5 Profitable and efficient production with emphasis on improved farm management and conservation of soil, water, energy, and biological resources.

Some examples of practices and principles emphasized in alternative systems include:

1 Crop rotations that mitigate weed, disease, insect, and other pest problems; increase available soil nitrogen and reduce the need for purchased fertilizers; and, in conjunction with conservation tillage practices, reduce soil erosion.
2 Integrated pest management, which reduces the need for pesticides by crop rotations, scouting, weather monitoring, use of resistant cultivars, timing of planting, and biological pest controls.
3 Management systems to control weed and improve plant health and the abilities of crops to resist insect pests and disease.
4 Soil- and water-conserving tillage.
5 Animal production systems that emphasize disease prevention through health maintenance, thereby reducing the need for antibiotics.
6 Genetic improvement of crops to resist insect pests and disease and to use nutrients more effectively.

The study, which monitored 14 successful organic farms over 5 years, concluded that 'well managed alternative farms use less synthetic chemicals, fertilisers, pesticides and antibiotics, without necessarily decreasing – and in some cases increasing – per acre crop yields and the productivity of livestock systems. Wider adoption of proven alternative systems would result in ever greater economic benefits to farmers and environmental gains for nations.' One of the farms included in the study had not used chemicals for 15 years and had corn yields 32% higher than the local average and soya bean yields 40% higher[321].

This was a very selective study of a small number of successful farms, and did not cover those that had tried organic methods and failed. Successful organic farming is likely to require greater management skills, longer working hours, and more varied work from farmers. The report observes that American farmers may not have the skills, the patience or the inclination to change their practices. Fewer than 5% (100000) of America's two million farmers use organic methods, while in the UK the figure is between 1000 and 1500. Consumer demand for 'organic food' is growing rapidly in both countries, leaving a shortfall in supply which has to be imported from abroad. Conversion to organic methods is a difficult and costly exercise, involving restructuring of farming practices which may take several years to achieve. Crop yields initially decline when chemicals are no longer used. Present indications are, that if organic farming is to be encouraged, there must be government incentive schemes, such as the conversion grants offered in Sweden, to help farmers through these initial difficult years. In January 1990 the UK government announced a system of subsidies, using European Community funds to give grants to farmers converting to organic agriculture.

Consumer demand for 'organic food' is growing rapidly.

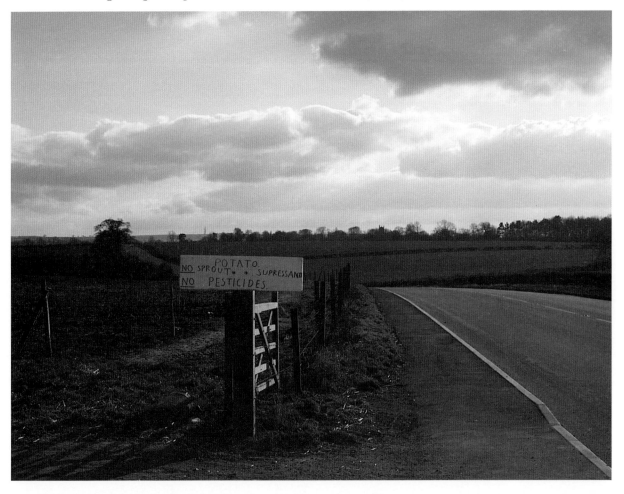

10 PESTICIDES IN THE NEXT CENTURY

It is a measure of the extent of professional and public concern that in 1988 the British Medical Association Board of Science and Education was asked to set up a Working Party to study the possible effects of pesticides on human health. The degree of public awareness of the pesticides issue is reflected in a survey conducted by the Department of the Environment in 1990[1] which showed that almost 80% of those polled were concerned about the present levels of pesticides, fertilizers and other chemicals in use.

This report examines the need for the current use of pesticides, reviews the literature concerning acute and chronic effects on human health, and the present methods of control and surveillance and considers the alternatives to chemical pesticides. Having reviewed the current situation, it is necessary to look forward to future action and development. What, in the opinion of the BMA, is the appropriate role for pesticides in the year 2000 and beyond?

PESTICIDES: EVALUATING THE RISK

Public perception of risk depends on many factors, such as whether the damage is acute or chronic, whether it affects individuals or society and whether the taking of risks is voluntary or involuntary. A hazard that is faced by choice, such as mountain climbing, is viewed with less alarm than an involuntary risk such as death by terrorist violence. Pesticides are an obvious focus for public concern because they are chemicals that are purposely released into the environment for the eradication of living organisms. In most circumstances, human exposure to pesticides is an involuntary risk, as humans may be exposed to pesticide residues in the food that they eat and the water they drink. Given the extensive use of pesticides for agricultural and non-agricultural purposes, most of the population probably have low-level exposure to pesticide residues in tap water. A report on a London-wide Survey of drinking water quality published by the Association of London Chief Environmental Health Officers found that no supplies were completely unaffected by herbicide residues[322]. Although there was no immediate risk to health, the report suggested that users of pesticides should consider changing to more environmentally acceptable alternatives where possible.

Any judgement about the extent to which the benefits outweigh possible risks from pesticides can never be a purely scientific matter, although it should be based on reliable and validated scientific data. However, to many people it appears that the British regulatory system operates on the assumption that these questions are purely technical matters which are best dealt with by expert committees, meeting in secret. While it may be right and proper that key decisions affecting the public good are delegated to individuals with specialist knowledge, responsibility cannot be surrendered completely to the expert committees. Even if we knew precisely how safe or toxic particular chemicals are, that by itself would not enable us to decide what level of risk is socially acceptable. Balancing risks against benefits involves making social judgements as well as scientific ones.

The information that has been reviewed in the preparation of this report has been extensive, although it has not been and could not be exhaustive. There is considerable – if incomplete – data on acute accidental and deliberate poisoning by pesticides worldwide. The number of deaths from accidental poisoning is particularly marked in developing countries, which tend to have fewer regulations governing manufacture and use. In the UK, there have been a small number of cases of acute toxicity, although it is expected that the figure is conservative due to under-reporting. With regard to chronic or long-term effects, the data are less conclusive. While no causal link has been proven between pesticides and forms of cancer, nervous and allergic diseases and reproduction problems, there are serious doubts about the scientific validity of some of the studies that have been undertaken and there is no epidemiological evidence available for many pesticides. In other words, we do not know whether many pesticides are harmful or not in day-to-day use. This lack of information clearly needs to be corrected, although data will be difficult to obtain. Given this uncertainty, it is difficult to make categorical statements on the degree of risk posed by pesticides, particularly the risk presented to human health.

THE NEED FOR A PESTICIDES POLICY

Our study has revealed two important findings: firstly, the incompleteness of existing knowledge concerning the effects of pesticide exposure on human health; and, secondly, the lack of a central strategy governing the use of pesticides. A pesticides policy would provide central guidance on desired levels of use, a review of measures of control and surveillance, as well as the research and development of alternatives to chemical pesticides. An active research programme is necessary to extend our knowledge of the likely effects of chemical pesticides on human health and to expand the limits of what it is possible to know. Direction from the government in the form of a national policy would enable a rational assessment of the future role of pesticides in food production, rather than a piecemeal or market-led strategy as at present. The Association believes there is a clear need for a national pesticides policy in this country, and the White Paper *This Common Inheritance* addresses this issue[323].

There are five key areas that could be addressed by a pesticides policy:

1 *Reduction* in the use of pesticides.
2 *Information*, in terms of new research and greater access to existing data so that informed decisions can be made by both responsible bodies and individual consumers.
3 *Diversification* of pest control methods.
4 *Regulation*, so that current testing, approval and enforcement measures are subject to review and improvement where possible.
5 *Education* of all those involved in the manufacture and application of the pesticides, as well as the doctors who may be expected to diagnose and treat symptoms of exposure to pesticides.

1 Reduction

Timetabled Reduction of Use
It is desirable that we should continue to decrease the use of conventional pesticides, where alternatives are available. A pesticides policy would feature a timetabled reduction of pesticides, as featured in the national pesticide policies of the Netherlands, West Germany and Scandinavia. Where chemical agents continue to be used, a phased reduction in the load applied would need to be implemented in conjunction with the development of better methods of application, so that smaller volumes of chemicals could be used more efficiently.

Minimal Use Strategy
The UK Government has already acknowledged the need for a judicious use of pesticides in the recent Code of Practice on Pesticides, produced jointly by the Ministry of Agriculture, Fisheries and Food and the Health and Safety Commission. This urged farmers to consider carefully the appropriate circumstances in which pesticides should be used; the farmer should have identified the particular pest that it is necessary to eliminate from a particular crop before the decision to use a chemical treatment is made. The Code states definitely that, 'Pesticides should only be used when necessary, in relation to efficient production, if the consequences of not using them significantly outweigh the risks to human health and the environment of using them.' This precautionary approach – a change of emphasis whereby the question 'why not use pesticides?' is replaced by the question 'why use pesticides?' – would form the central plank of a national pesticides policy.

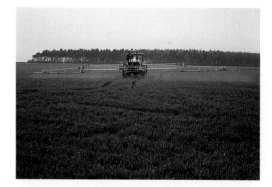

The farmer should have identified the particular pest before the decision to use chemical treatment is made.

2 Information

Information Strategy
A pesticides policy should have a two-pronged strategy on information: firstly, to make more accessible existing information; and, secondly, to commission and facilitate new research. There is also a need to improve the present mechanisms of collecting information on pesticide incidents for epidemiological purposes. Lack of information about how to gain access to data is perhaps the single greatest deficiency that has been identified by the British Medical Association with regards to

pesticides safety. Existing information must be brought into the public domain and greater efforts should be made to obtain more complete and comprehensive toxicological, epidemiological and other scientific data on chemical pesticides and their effects on human health.

Freedom of Information

Professional and public confidence in the regulation of pesticides depends largely on confidence in the quality of the scientific information upon which decisions are based. One of the hallmarks of good science is the open availability of information; therefore a defensible approach to the regulation of pesticides must rely upon information that is publicly available and subject to peer scrutiny and review.

Freedom of information legislation covering all chemicals is required, which would give adequate protection to commercial interests while providing access to data to legitimate enquirers. Under current law, pesticide manufacturers are required to provide sufficient information to demonstrate the safety of their products – within reasonable limits of human error – to the satisfaction of an official committee composed of independent experts; public access to these data should be improved. It should be noted that the case for freedom of information applies as much to the toxicological dossiers of compounds that are already licensed for use as it does to the dossiers on new compounds.

Open access to information about pesticides includes the provision of adequate information at the point of purchase and consumption of foodstuffs. The public have a right to know whether pesticides have been used during production or post-harvest storage. A system of food labelling which would indicate that pesticides had been used on that food product is highly desirable; a recent survey by MAFF of 1000 consumers showed that 50% wanted to know whether pesticides had been used in production of the food[324]. The public is also entitled to reassurance that *acceptable daily intakes*, which are based on the best toxicological data available, are not being exceeded. This will require more testing of either the basic crop or the food product.

Research and Development

In 1987 the Chairman's report of the House of Commons Select Committee on Agriculture said that he found the '. . . lack of epidemiological research quite unsatisfactory' and he urged the government to exert themselves to remedy that situation[2]. Research protocols in this area are difficult to design and implement but in 1990 there is no published evidence that steps have been taken to implement that recommendation effectively. There is an urgent need for concerted efforts by the Agricultural and Food Research Council (AFRC), the Medical Research Council, the Ministry of Agriculture, Food and Fisheries (MAFF), the Health and Safety Executive (HSE) and the Departments of Health and other interested bodies to resolve this problem.

A significant expansion of international research is required to improve and validate toxicological models. Only then will it be possible to estimate the validity of current methods of research and the way in which extrapolations can reasonably be made from the animal model, as predictors of human ill health.

The health of groups who are exposed to relatively high levels of pesticides through their work should be monitored closely.

One of the priorities for epidemiological work should be to monitor the health of groups who are exposed to relatively high levels of pesticide in the course of their employment, such as agricultural and forestry workers. Once the use of a pesticide compound or formulation has been approved there should be effective post-marketing surveillance. Comprehensive data are needed on the quantities of compounds in use and where, when and how such chemicals are applied, so that an accurate picture of current levels of exposure can be established. Data from such work are necessary for adequate epidemiological and environmental studies.

Our evidence suggests that there is insufficient information regarding the levels of pesticide residues in the national diet, and further research would improve our understanding of the complex interactions between pesticides and the natural components of foods, especially grains. Research is necessary to assess the extent of pesticide residues in both typical and extreme diets. To this end, an enhanced programme of residue monitoring by government laboratories is necessary.

Farmers, pesticide and farm machinery manufacturers and the Health and Safety Executive have already recognized the importance of applications technology but more research is needed into better methods of applying chemical pesticides. Better technical and engineering control over the handling and application of pesticides should replace the present over-reliance on personal protective clothing for operators. The use of design technology should be extended to improve the quality of packaging with the development of better forms of child-proof container, especially for pesticides sold for use in the home and garden.

Collating Information

To enhance the current state of knowledge, it is necessary to improve the present mechanism for collecting and reporting incidences of pesticide exposure. Two measures are necessary to achieve this end; the creation of a 'green card' reporting system in medical practice and a new central Pesticides Incident Monitoring Unit (PIMU).

The green card system should be analogous to the yellow card system, which is currently used to gather information about adverse reactions to pharmaceutical products. Under this arrangement, doctors and workers could and should report evidence of adverse effects to a central monitoring point; this reporting centre should be the new Pesticides Incident Monitoring Unit (PIMU) (Figure 10.1).

The PIMU would replace current arrangements under which several agencies collect data in an uncoordinated fashion. This should cover data from all groups who are exposed to pesticides, whether in employment, recreation or as third parties in cases of accidental exposure. The PIMU should work in close collaboration with such bodies as the Department of Health, the Health and Safety Executive, the Public Health Laboratory Service, Environmental Health Officers from local authorities and Directors of Public Health from district health authorities. Reports of the PIMU should be made available annually. The development of a national pesticide incident monitoring scheme would establish the scale of pesticide related problems in the UK more accurately.

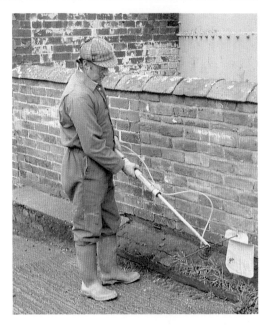

Better technical and engineering control over the handling and application of pesticides would afford greater protection to the worker.

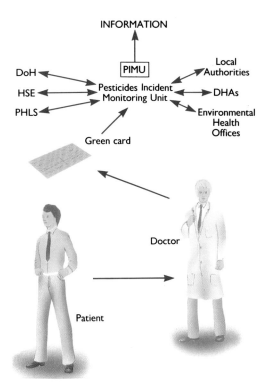

Figure 10.1
A new system of reporting pesticide-related illness has been proposed, which would improve the present mechanisms for collecting data on pesticide exposure incidents in the UK.

3 Diversification

Integrated Pest Management

We would like to see the development of an integrated pest management (IPM) scheme in the UK. An integrated pest management strategy would attempt to stabilise pest populations, maintaining them at tolerable levels instead of aiming to eradicate pests by blanket chemical control. For some time there would remain a need to eradicate certain pests by the minimal use of pesticides and very precise methods of application. Complementary, alternative methods should be deployed as soon as possible. Support should be provided to enable farmers to reduce their use of, and reliance upon, conventional pesticides.

Developing Alternatives

Alternatives to chemical pesticide use promoted by the EC and recent initiatives by the UK Government are welcome. One of the most constructive ways in which help could be given to organic, and lower input, farming would be by providing public support for appropriate research and development. This should focus on maintaining and improving soil fertility, on animal and plant breeding, on ways to maintain and improve pest resistance in crops and herds. MAFF and the Agricultural and Food Research Council (AFRC) should support a national programme of research and development to encourage investment into alternative technologies for weed, pest and disease control. More research is also needed on the ways in which pesticide and herbicide resistant varieties arise, with a view to developing strategies to avoid the pesticide treadmill.

4 Regulation

The Need for Reform

There is agreement among some experts that it is desirable and necessary to reform the regulatory system covering pesticides in Britain. Pesticides are regulated by the Minister of Social Services, Employment, Environment and MAFF, the HSE and the Scottish and Welsh offices as advised by the Advisory Committee on Pesticides (ACP). The ACP is comprised of independent experts and in turn, is supported by another independent group, the Scientific Sub-Committee, which actually evaluates all aspects of pesticide safety, including human and environmental matters.

However, a major weakness in the present regulatory system is the conflict of interest inherent in MAFF trying to regulate food production as well as pesticide safety. The Association believes that an independent Ministry of Food is essential and would clearly demonstrate the Government's commitment to the interests of the food consumer.

The need for greater freedom of information has been mentioned already; nowhere is this more marked than in the area of regulation of pesticides. The evaluation of applications for permission to market pesticides should be made more open and publicly accountable. In particular, the process by which decisions are made should be open to public scrutiny.

Protecting the Workers

It is recognized that a number of acute cases of pesticide poisoning occur owing to poor training, supervision or inadequate protective clothing for operators. The health and safety of workers responsible for the manufacture and application of pesticides should be improved. The Control of Substances Hazardous to Health Regulations (COSHH) 1988 are welcome in reinforcing the duty of the employer to implement proper control measures in the workplace.

In addition, agricultural, horticultural and forestry workers should enjoy the same legal health and safety rights as other sectors of the workforce. This is not the case at present; workers in agriculture, horticulture and forestry often do not have the opportunity to appoint Safety Representatives to monitor health and safety issues. These areas require rigorous health and safety representation because of the hazardous chemicals and equipment that are used; agriculture is judged to be the second or third most dangerous industry in terms of industrial accidents and deaths. A safer working environment for those in agriculture, horticulture and forestry would not only protect the workforce in these areas but also increase the level of protection for the public.

Approval and Registration

At present, there is a dual standard operating whereby the toxicological database for some of the older pesticides is less comprehensive than that of the newer compounds. The announcement by MAFF of its decision to undertake a complete review of older pesticides is welcome; sufficient resources should be made available by Her Majesty's Government for this review to be achieved within a reasonable time.

Permission should be granted for the introduction of new compounds, and approval renewed for previously permitted pesticides, only if they have advantages for human health over methods and products that are already available.

Testing Food and Water

The requirements for testing pesticides in food and water need to be developed further. Although they are already elaborate, they do not necessarily resolve important questions concerning possible hazards to public health and the environment.

We are concerned that not enough is known about the extent to which pesticides remain in foods and contaminate tap water. There are different methods that can be used to measure pesticide residues. Manufacturing industries should make available to the appropriate authorities their own analytical techniques for identifying trace concentrations of pesticide chemicals. There is need for more research to improve and validate the methods used for detecting and measuring pesticide residues.

It is of some concern that the UK does not yet have a comprehensive set of Maximum Residue Levels (MRLs) for all pesticides in foods. A comprehensive and defensible set of MRLs for all applied chemicals in all agricultural products should be established, in the UK and throughout the European Community, supported by a Community-wide as well as a comprehensive national residue testing system.

Similar problems of test methodologies and sampling arise in relation to tap water supplies. Contamination of ground-water by agricultural chemicals is becoming a major environmental concern; this is particularly worrying given that ground-water is the major source of drinking water in certain parts of the country. The Government should withhold approval for any pesticide that is likely to contaminate drinking water supplies, unless the manufacturer can specify an analytical method that is sufficiently sensitive to detect the compound at the appropriate level of concentration in tap water.

Review of Hazardous Practices
Investigations should be undertaken into particularly hazardous practices and techniques in the application of pesticides. There should be a thorough review of the risks and benefits of, and alternatives to, the aerial spraying of pesticides; the practice needs to be controlled more carefully than at present. In particular, we would like to see the system of public notification substantially improved, so that particularly vulnerable patient groups, such as those suffering from respiratory problems, may be alerted in advance of spraying activities.

One area that has caused particular concern is the use of 'total weedkillers' for non-agricultural purposes. A review, commissioned jointly by MAFF, the Department of the Environment and the Department of Health should be set up regarding the use of these chemicals by bodies such as British Rail, local authorities and industry. The impact of this practice on public health and the environment should be analysed in a comprehensive fashion, and the results of that study should be published.

Our report has drawn attention to shortcomings in controls on post-harvest pesticide treatments. We would like to eliminate what the MAFF Research Consultative Committee referred to in their 1989 report as 'bucket and shovel methods'. An enhanced system of control over post-harvest treatments should be established, and a detailed study of such methods of treatment should be undertaken and published.

International Standards
The completion of the single European market in 1992 is leading to European legislation which will govern pesticide regulations throughout the European Community. However, the harmonization of health, safety and environmental standards for pesticides could result in a lowering of standards to the level of the most poorly regulated state as the norm. Uniformly high standards of regulatory enforcement are vital, especially as the reduction of border controls after 1992 will allow agricultural commodities and processed foods to be distributed in an unrestricted fashion throughout the Community.

There is concern about the high incidence of acute poisoning from pesticides worldwide, especially in developing countries. The reasons for this may include poor packaging, labelling and training in the use of pesticides. There is a very real temptation for those in debt-ridden countries to use cheaper and possibly more hazardous compounds as an immediate solution to a food supply problem. The efforts of industries and governments worldwide to ensure that the regulations affecting pesticide safety do not simply apply to the wealthier developed countries must be coordinated.

Inspection

No set of regulations can be any more effective than the associated policing arrangements. For this reason we believe that a sufficient number of properly trained, qualified and equipped inspectors are necessary to ensure that regulations are enforced. The Institution of Professional and Civil Servants, which represents HSE inspectors, has stated that at least 100 extra Health and Safety Inspectors are essential for the proper enforcement of the relevant legislations.

5 Education

Educating the Doctors

General practitioners and hospital doctors have an important role to play in providing guidance to the public and patients about the hazards of toxic chemicals. They can, however, only fulfil their responsibilities if they receive sufficient training to enable them to recognize the symptoms of exposure to toxic chemicals when they encounter them. While it is sometimes difficult to identify cases of exposure to pesticides, given the non-specific nature of the symptoms, it is evident that the training available to doctors on these matters could be improved.

The training of medical students in the basics of toxicology should be given a higher priority than at present. Doctors who have completed their training should also have access to in-service education which would enable them to update and refresh their existing toxicological knowledge.

Training the Workers

The training of operators in the safe handling and application of chemical pesticides has already been noted as a requirement under the Control of Substances Hazardous to Health (COSHH) Regulations 1988. All operators should be trained in the proper handling of the application equipment they have to use. Some will need extra training in special operations, such as mixing pesticides for use or applying pesticides at reduced volumes.

All users, both employers and operators, need to continue to receive training that gives them up-to-date knowledge of all aspects of pesticide use, including legislation, the hazards posed by pesticides, safe working practices, emergency action in case of accidental exposure and the need for health surveillance and record keeping.

Since preparation of this report the World Health Organisation in collaboration with the United Nations Environment Programme has published a comprehensive report on pesticides revealing that 'the situation is particularly worrying in view of the lack of reliable data on the long-term consequences of exposure to pesticides.' They recommend better training and supervision of workers, improved legislation with more enforcement and long-term exposure studies for the general population[38].

PESTICIDES: THE PRECAUTIONARY APPROACH

Nothing in life is free of risk. When something is judged to be 'safe' it merely falls within acceptable limits of risk. In particular, chemical pesticides are not risk free. Action needs to be taken to ensure that the benefits arising from the use of chemical pesticides are not compromised by inadequate enforcement of existing regulations and ignorance of safe working procedures.

This report has reviewed a considerable quantity of evidence concerning pesticides, their safety and toxicity. The best strategy for dealing with these substances, where we are confronted by profound uncertainties and the need to set benefits against risks, is firstly to act cautiously, and secondly to embark on a systematic programme of research to improve our understanding.

The BMA endorses the principle that until we have a more complete understanding of pesticide toxicity, the benefit of the doubt should be awarded to protecting the environment, the worker and the consumer. More particularly, where there are serious concerns relating to the safety of a particular pesticide, its use should be withdrawn or restricted until a new risk/benefit analysis can be made. The continuing use of the particular pesticide must then be related to the degree of uncertainty and the potential severity of effects for human health. This precautionary approach is necessary because the data on risk to human health from exposure to pesticides are incomplete.

An effective pesticides strategy combines the discipline of science and the value of prudence, qualities that the medical profession aims to foster in the maintenance of the nation's public and environmental health.

APPENDIX

There are a number of courses and examinations available in the UK which offer training and professional qualifications in toxicology. Listed below are major examples.

MRCPath EXAMINATION

The Royal College of Pathologists (RCPath) provide examinations in toxicology and other subjects.

The MRCPath examination is divided into Parts I and II.

For Part I, candidates must have worked in a recognised training department for at least three years, of which two and a half years must have been in toxicology. There are elements of training common to all disciplines such as the introduction of the trainee to matters of administration, management, budget control, health and safety at work, quality assurance, data processing and the use of computers.

If possible, involvement in undergraduate teaching and participation in postgraduate training by attendance at departmental and interdepartmental meetings with clinicians, journal clubs and Clinical Pathological Conference (CPCs) would be advantageous. Candidates should be familiar with the scientific advances in their speciality. Attendance at postgraduate specialised courses and the acquisition of relevant MScs and other postgraduate qualifications should be encouraged.

Those wishing to take Part II of the examination must have completed five years full-time approved training, two years of which must have been in posts recognised for higher specialist training and four years in the branch of pathology chosen for the examination.

Further details may be obtained from the Royal College of Pathologists, 2 Carlton House Terrace, London SW1Y 5AF.

DIPLOMATE OF THE INSTITUTE OF BIOLOGY IN TOXICOLOGY (DIBT)

The Institute of Biology offer a postgraduate diploma examination in toxicology.

Students must have an honours science degree in an appropriate subject or subjects, plus five years' experience in an appropriate institution together with evidence of practical experience gained through participation or observation.

Nineteen different topic areas are covered including genetic toxicology, behavioural toxicology, immunotoxicology, ecotoxicology, radiation toxicology and clinical toxicology.

Candidates must sit three theory papers which test breadth

and depths of knowledge and then undertake either laboratory-based intensive research or a critical review of literature and present a dissertation of approximately 8000 words 10 months after the written examination.

Further details may be obtained from the Institute of Biology, 20 Queensberry Place, London SW7 2DZ.

The DIBT qualification may also be obtained through the Toxicology course offered by the North East Surrey College of Technology, see under Postgraduate Research Training and Other Courses.

HIGHER EDUCATION COURSES IN TOXICOLOGY

A number of UK higher education institutions offer degree or diploma courses in toxicology or related disciplines; places are open to part-time students. The following list is a guide to some of these courses but intending students should seek confirmation on availability and entrance requirements from the institution concerned.

University of Wales: Swansea

Genetic Toxicology
Diploma
Theoretical and practical aspects of the study and evolution of potentially hazardous chemical and physical agents; general toxicology, mutagenicity tests, *in vitro* and *in vivo* assays, foreign compound metabolism; biological effects of mutation. Examination.

University of Birmingham

Toxicology
MSc
Provides training in the theoretical and practical aspects of toxicity and comprises a research project and 5 modules (each of 5 weeks) in: the basis and significance of chemical induced toxicity; recognition and detection of acute and chronic toxicity; metabolism of xenobiotics; pharmacological aspects of toxicology; toxic hazards. Written examination and project report.

Toxicological Studies
Diploma
A programme of study with a broadly similar content to the MSc in toxicology. Primarily intended for students seconded from industry, those not intending to enter laboratory-based employment and as a possible preparation for PhD study.

University of Glasgow

Forensic Toxicology
MSc
Courses as for the diploma (below); further lectures dealing mainly with subjects other than chemistry (for example, pathology, law, interpretation); and a supervised project. Examination by written papers and dissertation.

Diploma
Lectures and seminars cover the field of analytical chemistry

applied to drugs, environmental contaminants and general chemicals in human tissue, and the interpretation of the results. Laboratory work includes all the techniques used in a modern analytical toxicology laboratory dealing with human tissue. Examination by written papers.

Diploma
Designed for lawyers, scientists, doctors and others involved in court work and court procedure. Lecture and seminars held on a weekday evenings and weekends. Includes forensic and general pathology; forensic toxicology; basic statistical evaluation of results; principals of law of evidence and procedure. Examination (written, oral and practical).

University of London: Royal Postgraduate Medical School

Experimental Pathology (Toxicology)
MSc
Course concerned with the biological response in humans to medicines and to toxic chemicals in the environment. Taught jointly by the departments of histopathology and clinical pharmacology. Coursework assessment examination (written, practical and oral) and report.

University of Surrey

Toxicology
MSc
Prepares suitable science, veterinary and medical graduates for careers in toxicology (in industry, government regulatory bodies or research establishments) by providing them with an understanding and appreciation of the many facets of the subject. Particular emphasis placed upon the molecular mechanisms of chemically induced toxicity. Continuous assessment examination (written and oral) and research project dissertation.

Aberdeen University

Clinical Pharmacology
MSc
A twelve month full-time course designed to give instruction in the specialist aspects of Clinical Pharmacology from both the laboratory and clinical aspects. A component in toxicology is included and research training in toxicology may be undertaken.

Hatfield Polytechnic

Pharmacological Biochemistry
MSc
A 2 year part-time course designed for graduates who have practical experience in fundamental aspects of drug action or who are involved in the design, screening and development of new drugs, as well as for graduates working within the NHS who are concerned with the use and effectiveness of drugs. In

the second year of the course a 42 lecture option may be taken in Biochemical and Predictive Toxicology.

Portsmouth Polytechnic

Applied Toxicology
MSc

A one year full-time course with the principle objective of equipping graduates with backgrounds in biology or biomedical sciences, or pharmacy, or chemistry for a career in toxicology in industrial and public sectors. Course topics include: A Foundation in the Industrial Background to Toxicology, Biochemical Toxicology, Cell and Tissue Toxicology, Analytical Techniques, Techniques for Bioassay, Data Analysis and Interpretation, and Legislation and Toxicology. The requirements of industry are of paramount importance in the continuing development of the philosophy of this degree.

North East London Polytechnic

Pharmacology
MSc

A two year day-release course designed so that graduates in appropriate biological subjects can obtain advanced training in Pharmacology and thereby become more effective in industry, research institutions and pharmacies. The toxicity of drugs and food additives forms part of the course syllabus.

POSTGRADUATE RESEARCH TRAINING AND OTHER COURSES

The North East Surrey College of Technology provides a course for scientists who have an interest and/or practical expertise in this field. It follows the syllabus recommended by the Institute of Biology in preparation for the Postgraduate Qualification in Toxicology examinations. There are no formal entry requirements for this course but candidates can if they wish sit the DIBT examinations at the end of the course. Candidates wishing to sit the Diplomate of the Institute of Biology in Toxicology (DIBT) examinations must register separately with the Institute of Biology whose entry qualifications will apply.

The British Industrial Biological Research Association offer postgraduate research training in toxicology.

St Bartholomew's Hospital Medical College also offer postgraduate research training in toxicology.

GLOSSARY

A

Acceptable daily intake (ADI)	The amount of a pesticide that can be ingested every day throughout a person's life with the high probability, based on the known facts, that no harm will result.
Acid rain	Atmospheric precipitation with a pH below 5.6–5.7. One cause of this is the burning of fossil fuels which generate oxides of nitrogen and sulphur which are converted into nitric and sulphuric acids and washed down in rain. Acid rain can cause erosion of stonework and interferes with forested ecosystems. It can also lead to the sterilization of lakes where it accumulates.
Active ingredient	The particular chemical that causes the desired effect.
Acute exposure	Sudden exposure which may have severe, short-term effects leading to recovery, chronic illness or death.
Adjuvant	Chemicals added to a pesticide eg sticking agents, surfactants, solvents, inerts to increase its efficiency.
Agrochemical	Chemicals used in the production, protection and use of crops and livestock.
Allergy	Altered immunological reactivity in humans and animals to allergens (substances foreign to the body) induced by exposure through injection, inhalation, ingestion or skin contact.
Ames test	A test in which special bacteria are used to assess whether a chemical will damage the genetic information (DNA) in cells and help predict whether the chemical may also by this means cause cancer.
Amine	Important type of organic compound.
Anabolic	Relating to, or promoting the process of making new living tissue from nutrient material.
Anaerobic biological denitrification	Denitrification process caused by the action of anaerobic bacteria.
Anencephaly	Absence of the brain due to an effect occurring during development.
Anthelmintic	A remedy for infestation with worms.

Antimicrobial	A substance which destroys bacteria or inhibits their growth.
Aphicides	Chemical to kill aphids.
Aplastic anaemia	Severe, fatal blood condition where the bone marrow has partially or completely ceased to function.
Aquatic biota	Combined flora and fauna living in water.
Aquifer	A water-bearing rock formation which may be porous, unconsolidated gravel, fractured rock, or cavernous limestone which yields economically important amounts of water to wells.
Aracicide	Chemical to kill spiders.
Atropine	An anti-cholinergic drug.

B

Bacteria	Single-celled microorganisms usually measuring 0.3–0.2 micrometres in diameter possessing the prokaryotic type of cell construction.
Bilharzia	Also *Schistosoma*. A genus of blood flukes. Adult parasites inhabit veins, laying eggs which pass into the small vessels of the intestine or bladder.
Bioaccumulation	The build-up of substances within the tissues of living organisms.
Bioassay	A method of determining the concentration or activity of a substance by testing it on a living organisms under controlled conditions.
Biochemical oxygen demand (BOD)	A measure of how readily an effluent, during the natural processes of oxidation to which it is subject, removes oxygen dissolved in the water of a river or stream.
Biocide	Chemical designed to kill a broad spectrum of pests, including fungus.
Biodegradable	Substance which is capable of being broken down by microorganisms.
Biological control	Method of regulating plant and animals pests by natural predators.
Biotechnology	Use of living cells or microorganisms in industry to manufacture drugs and chemicals, create energy, destroy waste matter, etc.
Bipyridils	Herbicides and dissicants eg paraquat and diquat.
Blue baby syndrome	A new-born child with a blue appearance of the skin due to deficient oxygenation of the blood (cyanosis): in the toxicological context, the appearance may be caused by methaemoglobinaemia.
Borehole	A bore in the earth's surface for investigation or for extraction of water, oil etc.
Brackish water	A mixture of fresh and salt water.

C

Carbamates	Synthetic insecticides containing carbon, sulphur and hydrogen eg bendiocarb and carbaryl.
Carcinogenicity	The ability of a substance/condition to produce or give rise to tumours.
Carrier	Liquid or solid substance added to a pesticide to facilitate application.
Catalytic converters	A device used for removing pollutant from automotive exhaust by promoting the chemical reactions for the conversion of these pollutants to carbon dioxide, water and nitrogen.
Cataracts	Opacity in the crystalline lens of the eye.
Chloracne	A widespread acneform eruption due to exposure to chlorinated naphthalenes, chlordiphenyls (better known as polychlorinated biphenyls), chlordiphenyl oxides and chlorinated dibenzodioxins and dibenzodifurans.
Cholinesterase	An enzyme present in the blood and tissues at the endings of voluntary motor nerves and nerves of the parasympathetic division of the involuntary system and synapses.
Chromosome	Chromosomes contain genes arranged in linear order along their length. The genetic information is carried in chromosomes in their DNA. Chromosomes are located in the nucleus in plant and animal cells.
Chronic	Long continued.
Co-carcinogen	A substance which can enhance the effects of a carcinogen.
Cohort	A group of individuals who have a common characteristic, often identified by the year of birth or exposure, who are studied over a long period of time.
Companion planting	Growing one crop alongside another so that its natural pest-repellent qualities will protect the other from damage. See intercropping.
Compounds	Chemical combination of two or more substances.
Congenital malformation	Abnormality of any portion or organ of the body that develops during pregnancy.
Controlled Droplet Application	A method of applying pesticides which causes less drift than from older hydraulic sprays.

Crop rotation	An agricultural system whereby different crops are grown in an area each season (including one season when the area is left fallow), so that the optimum condition of the soil is maintained.
Cross-resistance	The resistance that an organism develops to one substance and is able to use to resist the toxic effects of other similar chemicals. When this develops it is called the 'domino-effect'.
Cryptosporidium	A protozoan organism that infects the gastrointestinal tract of various animal species.
Cytotoxic	Damaging to cell structure and division.

D

Denitrification	The removal of nitrogen or its compounds.
Dessificant	Chemical which causes plants to dry out and wither eg paraquat.
Detergent swans	Large mobile aggregates of detergent bubbles which are not destroyed by normal sewage treatment occurring on rivers etc.
Dithiocarbamates	Insecticide group containing maneb, nabem and zineb.
Domino-effect	See cross-resistance.

E

EBDCs	See dithiocabarmates. Ethylenebisdithiocarbamate.
Ecosystem	A contraction of the term ecological system. A functional system which includes the organisms of a natural community together with their environment.
Emulsifiable concentrate (EC)	A homogeneous liquid formation which forms an emulsion on mixing with water.
Epidemiology	The science that investigates the causes of disease, often through the study of the distribution of diseases in particular population groups.
Eutrophication	The deterioration of the aesthetic and life-supporting qualities of lakes and estuaries, caused by excessive fertilization from effluents high in phosphorous, nitrogen and organic growth substances, leading to excessive growth of algae and aquatic plants.

Excipient	A binding or other agent enabling a chemical to be made into a medicine or other useful product eg a pesticide. An excipient will biologically have no medicinal properties of its own or be able to render the drug ineffective, as it is used to make the chemical more stable, more palatable or to give it better handling properties.

F

Fallowing	To leave agricultural land untilled or unsown for a time.
Fertilizer	Materials added to the soil, or applied directly to crop foliage, to supply elements needed for plant nutrition.
Flocculation	The gathering together of small particles dispersed in a solution to form larger particles.
Food chain	A series of organisms connected by the fact that each forms food for the next higher organism in the series.
Fossil fuel	Carbon-containing materials that are burned with air (or oxygen) to supply heat for any purpose. At normal temperatures these fuels can be solid eg coal, liquid eg oil, or gas eg natural gas.
Fungicide	Chemical compounds used to control plant diseases caused by fungi.
Fungus	One of a group of non-vascular plants which lack chlorophyll and whose reproductive and vegetative structures do not permit them to be included with algae or higher plants.

G

Genetic engineering	The preparation and joining together of two DNA molecules in a test tube and the subsequent insertion of this recombinant molecule into a living system. This method is used to produce organisms with beneficial characteristics which would not naturally occur or which only occur very rarely in nature.
Genotoxic carcinogens	Those substances which cause cancer by interfering with the genetic information in cells of animals.
Glioma	A tumour most commonly found in the brain but also in the spinal cord and occasionally in the roots of the cranial nerves.

Green card system	A proposed system for reporting pesticide incidents, similar to the existing 'Yellow card system' for adverse reactions to drugs.
Ground-water	Any liquid water residing beneath the surface of the earth.

H

Heavy metals	A metal of high specific atomic weight eg cadmium, copper, mercury, lead.
Herbicide	Any chemical used to destroy or inhibit plant growth, especially of weeds or other undesirable vegetation.
Hydrocarbons	One of a group of chemical compounds composed only of hydrogen and carbon. Natural sources include natural gas and petroleum. Hydrocarbons are also produced when coal is burnt.
Hydrosphere	The hydrosphere consists of all the water covering the surface of the earth (either liquid or solid) together with ground-waters.

I

Immune suppression	The natural or induced active suppression of the body's defence mechanism against infection and foreign substances (immune response).
Induced pest	An organism, not previously considered a pest until its predator (the original pest) is removed. It is then able to reproduce unhindered and becomes a pest in its own right.
Inorganic compounds	Compounds of any elements in the periodic table with the exception of the element carbon.
Insecticide	A material used to kill insects and related animals by disruption of vital processes through chemical action.
Integrated pest management (IPM)	The combination of traditional cultural methods, such as crop rotation, fallowing, the encouragement of natural predators etc, and modern chemical techniques.
Inter-haline zone	The area of transition between freshwater and seawater.
Intercropping	To grow or cultivate in alternate rows.
In vitro (tests)	Conducted on an artificial system not involving a living animal or plant eg a culture of cells in a test tube.
In vivo (tests)	Conducted on living animals.

| Ion | An atom, or group of atoms, which by loss or gain of one or more electrons has acquired an electric charge. |
| Ion exchange | Reversible exchanges of ions of the same charge sign between a solution (usually aqueous) and an insoluble solid in contact with it. |

L

Landfill	The disposal of waste into a hole in the ground.
Larvacide	Insecticide which controls larvae.
LD_{50}	The lethal dose which, when administered to a group of animals causes the death of 50% of those animals.
Leachate	Substances that migrate from a waste dump.
Lepeophtheirus salmonis	Parasitic salmon louse.
Listeria	A bacterium present in the environment, notably found in milk and milk products, infection by which in man may manifest as a meningoencephalitis.
Lymphoma	A group of malignant tumours, most commonly begun in the lymph nodes of the neck and underarm regions. As the disease progresses, so any organ in the body can become diseased. The liver, spleen and other lymph nodes are usually affected.

M

Maximum admissible concentration (MAC)	A measure of the maximum admissible concentration of a pesticide in water intended for human consumption which was introduced by a Council of Europe Directive (80/778/EEC).
Maximum residue levels (MRLs)	Maximum acceptable level of pesticide residue left in the crop.
Metabolism	The sum total of the chemical processes by which living organisms produce energy.
Methaemo-globinaemia	A derivative of haemoglobin in which the ferrous iron of haemoglobin is oxidized to ferric iron.
Microgram	1000 micrograms = 1 milligram.
Micron	One millionth of a metre; a micrometre.
Microorganisms	Either unicellular or multicellular small simple organisms, consisting of protozoa, algae, fungi, rickettsiae, viruses and bacteria. They are neither true plants nor animals.

Mildew	A fungal disease of plants.
Miscarriage	Abortion; expulsion of the foetus before it is viable.
Molluscicide	An agent for destroying molluscs eg snails, which eat crops.
Mutagenicity	The ability of a substance or condition to cause alteration of the genetic material of an organism, leading to inherited differences (mutation).
Myeloma	A locally malignant tumour, found most often at the end of long bones and in the jaw.

N

Neoplasm	A tumour.
Nervous system	The brain, spinal cord, and nerves collectively.
Neurotoxin	A substance poisonous to nerve tissue.
Nitrate	A salt of nitric acid, used as a fertilizer. It can be natural or synthetic.
Nitrogen cycle	The transformation process through which nitrogen and nitrogenous compounds pass in nature from free nitrogen to free nitrogen.
Non-degradable organic substance	A substance that is not broken down in soil or water.
No observed effect level (NOEL)	The highest dose at which no observable effects are detected, by any means, on laboratory animals.

O

Occupational exposure limits (OELs)	The maximum UK legal occupational exposure to chemicals.
Organic farming	An agricultural system that avoids or excludes the use of synthetic fertilizers and pesticides.
Organo-chlorine pesticides	A group of pesticides (such as DDT) containing one or more chlorine atoms; these can be very persistent.
Organo-phosphorous pesticides	A group of pesticides containing a phosphorous atom; they do not normally persist for long but can be very toxic.
Oxidation	The combining of oxygen with other molecules or an equivalent chemical change.

P

Parasite	An organism which lives on or in another organism and derives subsistence from it without rendering it any benefit in return.
Pathogenic organism	An organism that causes disease.
Pesticide	A material used for the mitigation, control, or elimination of plants or

	animals detrimental to human health or economy.
Petrochemicals	A large number of chemical substances produced commercially from petroleum or natural gas.
Phytoplankton	Microscopic algae which inhabit the illuminated surface waters of the sea, estuaries, lakes and ponds. Varieties include Diatoms and Dinoflagellates, found in marine, estuarine, and fresh-water environments and Coccolitho-phorids which do not occur in fresh water.
Pollution	Anything that contaminates or makes any feature of the environment offensive or harmful to human, animal or plant life.
Polychlorinated biphenyls (PCBs)	A generic term covering a family of partially or wholly chlorinated isomers of biphenyl. Sources include sewage outfalls, industrial and municipal disposal, leaking from dumps and burning of refuse.
Polymerization	The linking of small molecules to make larger molecules.
Polyneuropathy	A disease state in which a number of nerves are affected at the same time.
Potato blight	Fungus which caused devastation of the 1850s Irish potato crops.
Prior Informed Consent (PIC) Scheme	The method by which an exporting country intending to make a shipment of pesticides to another country secures the importing country's specific consent before shipment. The importing government should have full knowledge of the domestic regulatory status of the pesticide, including any bans or restrictions on its use.
Prophylactic	An agent or remedy used to prevent disease.
Pyrethroids	A group of selective insecticides which are structurally related to a class of naturally occurring pesticides.

R

Red List	As drawn up from EC Directive 76/464 it is a list of 22 chemicals and metals which because of their toxicity, persistence and potential for bioaccumulation of organisms in water, are considered priority pollutants in the UK.

S

Safener	Chemicals that reduce the potential of a pesticide to harm the crop itself.

Salmonella	A type of pathogenic bacterium which causes typhoid fever, paratyphoid fever and food poisoning in man.
Sarcoma	A malignant tumour of connective tissue or its derivatives.
Surfactant	A substance which exerts a marked effect on the surface behaviour of a system; eg the interface between solid–solid, solid–liquid, solid–gas, liquid–liquid or liquid–gas.
Suspension concentrate (SC)	A stable suspension of finely ground active ingredient(s) in a fluid intended for dilution before use.
Synthetic chemicals	Artificially produced chemicals like, and which can be a substitute for, natural chemicals.

T

Taenia saginata	The beef tapeworm. The adult form is parasitic to man.
Teratogenicity	The ability of a substance or condition to cause deviations from the normal growth and development between conception and birth, resulting in abnormal individuals.
Threshold limit values (TLVs)	The maximum legal occupational exposure limits in the USA (see OELs for UK limits).
Toxicity	A measure of a substance's ability to cause harm and the nature of that harm.
Toxicology	The study of harmful effects of chemicals on living systems.
Toxin	A specific poison of biological organic origin.

V

Vector	A carrier of disease or infection.
Virus	An infective agent consisting only of nucleic acid which may be encased in a protein shell. The largest measures only a few hundred-thousandths of an inch.

W

Weeds	Any plant growing where it is not wanted by man.

Y

Yellow card system	A yellow card which is used by doctors in the UK to report adverse drug reactions to the Committee on Safety of Medicines of the Department of Health.

REFERENCES

1. Central Statistical Office. *Social Trends 1990.* London: HMSO, 1990.
2. Agriculture Committee of the House of Commons. *The Effects of Pesticides on Human Health. Vol I Report and Proceedings of the Committee. Vol II Minutes of Evidence. Vol III Appendices to Minutes of Evidence.* Second Special Report. Session 1986–87. London: HMSO 1987.
3. Royal Commission on Environmental Pollution. *Agriculture and Pollution* Seventh Report. (Cmnd 7644). London: HMSO, 1979.
4. Department of the Environment. *The Nitrate Issue.* London: HMSO, 1988.
5. *Agriculture Encyclopaedia Britannica.* Chicago: William Benton, 1967.
6. Crone, H. D. *Chemicals and Society: A Guide to the New Chemical Age.* Cambridge: Cambridge University Press, 1986.
7. Thomas, K. *Religion and the Decline of Magic.* Harmondsworth: Penguin, 1973.
8. Bushaway, B. *By Rite: Custom, Ceremony and Community in England 1700–1880.* London: Junction Books, 1982.
9. Defoe, D. *A Tour Through the Whole Island of Great Britain.* Harmondsworth: Penguin, 1971.
10. Ashton, T. S. *An Economic History of England: The Eighteenth Century.* London: Methuen, 1972.
11. Tyler, A. *Street Drugs.* London: New English Library, 1986.
12. Hassall, K. A. *The Chemistry of Pesticides.* London: Macmillan, 1982.
13. Friend, G. The potential for a sustainable agriculture. In Knorr, D. (ed.) *Sustainable Food Systems.* Chichester: Ellis Horwood, 1983.
14. *Famine: The Irish Experience 900–1900.* Edinburgh: J. Donald, 1989.
15. Martin, H. *The Scientific Principles of Plant Protection with Special Reference to Chemical Control.* London: Arnold, 1928.
16. Carson, R. *The Silent Spring.* Harmondsworth: Penguin, 1985.
17. Goldsmith E. and Hildyard N. (eds). *Green Britain or Industrial Wasteland?* Cambridge: Polity, 1986.
18. Cazeneuve, P. Sur les dangers de l'emploi des insecticides à base aresenicale en agriculture au point de vue de l'hygiene publique. *Bulletin de L'Academic de Medicine, Paris* 1908; **lix**, 133–54.
19. Cramer, H. H. Plant protection and world food production. *Pflanzenschutz-nachrichten Bayer* 1967; **20(1)**, 7–517.
20. Groupement International des Associations Nationales de Fabricants de Produits Agrochemiques. *Pesticide Residues in Food.* Brussels: GIFAP, 1985.
21. United Nations Food and Agriculture Organisation. *Agriculture: Towards 2000* (C79/24). Rome: FAO, 1979.

22. Vogtmann, H. *The Quality of Agricultural Produce Originating from Different Systems of Cultivation*. Bristol: Soil Association, 1981.

23. Ministry of Agriculture, Fisheries and Food. *Report of the Working Party on Pesticide Residues: 1985–88*. The twenty-fifth report of the Steering Group on Food Surveillance. Food Surveillance Paper No 25. London: HMSO, 1989.

24. Roberts, M. B. U. *Biology: A Functional Approach*. London: Nelson, 1971.

25. Tivey, J. and O'Hare, G. *Human Impact on the Ecosystem*. Edinburgh: Oliver and Boyd, 1981.

26. Knight A. L., and Norton, G. W. Economics of agricultural pesticides resistance in arthropods. *Annual Review of Entomology* 1989; **34**, 293–313.

27. Bhantnagar, P., and Kumar, S. Update and bioconcentration of dieldrin, dimethoate and permethrin by *Tetrahymena pyriformis. Water, Air and Soil Pollution* 1989; **40**, 345–9.

28. Felsot, A. S. Enhanced biodegradation of insecticides in soil: implications for agroecosystems. *Annual Review of Entomology* 1989; **34**, 453–6.

29. Felsot, A. S. *Annual Review of Entomology* 1989; **34**, 753–6.

30. Rubin, B. Effect of Monoculture on Herbicide Efficacy. *Phytoparasitica* 1988; **16**, 359–60.

31. Audus, L. J. The biological detoxication of 2:4 dichlorophenoxyacetic acid in soil. *Plant and Soil* 1949; **2**, 31–6.

32. Agricultural Science Service. *Research & Development Report*, 275(85). London: MAFF, 1985.

33. Dover, M. and Croft, B. *Getting Tough: Public Policy and the Management of Pesticide Resistance*. Washington DC: World Resources Institute, 1984.

34. Gressel, J. Evolution of weeds with multiple herbicide resistances: a new problem with dire consequences. *Phytoparasitica* 1988; **16**, 364.

35. Metcalf, R. L. Insect resistance to insecticides. *Pesticides Science* 1989; **26**, 333–58.

36. Dudley, N. *The Poisoned Earth: The Truth About Pesticides*. London: Piatkus, 1987.

37. International Agency for Research on Cancer. *Monograph on the Evaluation of the Carcinogenic Risk of Chemicals to Humans*. Vol. 30, *Miscellaneous Pesticides*. Lyons: IARC, 1983.

38 World Health Organisation *Public health impact of pesticides used in agriculture*. Geneva; WHO, 1990.

39. Coggon, D. Are pesticides carcinogenic? *British Medical Journal* 1987; **294**, 725.

40. Ministry of Agriculture, Fisheries and Food. *Research Consultative Committee, Residues Sub-Group Report*. London; MAFF, 1989.

41. Bull, D. *A Growing Problem: Pesticides and the Third World Poor*. Oxford: Oxfam, 1982.

42. Holmes, J. Nitrate or new dawn? *Town and Country Planning*. 1987; **56**, 131–2.

43. Hodges, D. Agriculture, nitrates and health. *Soil Association Quarterly Review* 1985; **September**, 16–18.

44. Royal Society. *The Nitrogen Cycle of the United Kingdom.* London: Royal Society, 1983.

45. Ryan, J. A. *et al.* Plant uptake of non-ionic organic chemicals from soils. *Chemosphere* 1988; **17**, 2299–2323.

46. Van der Hoeven, A. Mutagenicity of extracts of some commonly consumed vegetables in the Netherlands. *Journal of Agriculture and Food Chemistry* 1983; **31**, 1020–6.

47. Goldsmith, E. and Hidlyard, N. (eds.) *The Earth Report: Monitoring the Battle for our Environment.* London: Mitchell Beazley, 1988.

48. Hester, R. E. *Understanding our environment.* London: Royal Society of Chemistry, 1986.

49. World Health Organisation. *Drinking Water Quality: Guidelines for Selected Herbicides.* Environmental Health, No. 27, WHO 1987.

50. Lees, A. and McVeigh, K. *An Investigation of Pesticide Pollution in Drinking Water in England and Wales.* London: Friends of the Earth, 1988.

51. Hellawell, J. Toxic substances in rivers and streams. *Environmental Pollution,* 1988; **50**, 61–85.

52. British Geological Survey. *The Pollution Threat from Agricultural Pesticides and Industrial Solvents.* London: BGS, 1987.

53. Craig, F. and Craig, P. *Britain's Poisoned Water.* Harmondsworth: Penguin, 1989.

54. Working Party on Pesticides Residues. *Anabolic, Anthelminthic and Antimicrobial Agents.* Food Surveillance Paper No. 22. London: HMSO, 1988.

55. Lashford, S. *The Residue Report.* Wellingborough: Thorsons, 1988.

56. Price, B. *Friends of the Earth Guide to Pollution.* London: Maurice Temple Smith, 1983.

57. Organisation for Economic Co-operation and Development. *Eutrophication of Waters: Monitoring, Assessment and Control.* Paris: OECD, 1982.

58. The Lowermoor Incident Health Advisory Group *Water Pollution at Lowermoor North Cornwall.* Truro: Cornwall and Isles of Scilly District Health Authority, 1989.

59. Martyn, C. N., *et al.* Geographical relation between Alzheimer's disease and aluminium in drinking water. *Lancet* 1989; **i**, 59–62.

60. Department of the Environment. *Lead in the environment.* Pollution Paper No 19. London: HMSO, 1983.

61. MAFF. *Lead in food: Progress Report, the Twenty Seventh Report of the Steering Group on Food Surveillance, the Working Party on Organic Contaminants in Food, Third Supplementary Report on Lead.* Food surveillance paper No. 27. London: HMSO, 1989.

62. World Health Organisation. *Guidelines for Drinking-Water Quality. Vol. 1 Recommendations.* Geneva: WHO, 1984.

63. Topp, E. Factors Affecting the Uptake of ^{14}C – labelled organic chemicals by plant by soil. *Ecotoxicology and Environmental Safety.* 1986; 11, 219–28.

64. Finney, J. *Demisting the Crystal Ball: World Crop Protection Prospects.* Haslemere: ICI Agrochemicals, 1988.

65. US Department of Health, Education and Welfare: National Institute for Occupational Safety and Health. *Occupational Exposure During the Manufacture and Formulation of Pesticides.* Washington DC: NIOSH, 1978.

66. US Department of Health, Education and Welfare: National Institute for Occupational Safety and Health. *Proceedings of the NIOSH Symposium on Health Hazard Control in the Pesticide Formulating and Manufacturing Industry, December 1980, St Louis, Missouri.* New York: Dialogue Systems, 1980.

67. Sittig, M. *Pesticides Manufacturing and Toxic Control Encyclopedia.* New Jersey: Noyes, 1980.

68. Whorton, D. *et al.* Infertility in male pesticide workers *Lancet* 1977; **ii**, 1259–61

69 Roberts, H. A. *Weed Control Handbook* (7th edn). Oxford: Blackwell, 1982.

70. Ministry of Agriculture, Fisheries and Foods. *Data Requirements for Approval Under the Control of Pesticides Regulations 1986.* London: MAFF, 1986.

71. Hay, A. Toxic cloud over Seveso. *Nature (Lond.)* 1976; **262**, 636–8.

72. Hay, A. *The Chemical Scythe: Lessons of 2,4,5-T and Dioxin.* London: Plenum, 1982.

73. Cook, J. and Kaufman, C. *Portrait of a Poison: the 2,4,5-T Story.* London: Pluto Press, 1982.

74. Margerison, T., *et al. Superpoison.* London: Macmillan, 1980.

75. Mastroiacovo, M. D. *et al.* Birth defects in the Seveso area after TCDD contamination. *Journal of the American Medical Association* 1988; **259**, 1668–72.

76. Department of the Environment. *Dioxins in the Environment.* Report of an Interdepartmental Working Group on polychlorinated dibenzo-para-dioxins (PCDDs) and polychlorinated dibernzofurans (PCDFs). Pollution Paper No. 27. London: HMSO, 1989.

77. Water Exchange and Pollution in the North Sea. Hamburg: University of Hamburg, 1989.

78. Health and Safety Executive. *Guidance Note CS19 Storage of Approved Pesticides* and *Pesticides.* Agricultural Safety Leaflet 27. London: HSE, 1988.

79. United Nations Food and Agriculture Organisation. *International Code of Conduct on the Distribution and Use of Pesticides.* Rome: FAO, 1986.

80. Geach, N. G. E. The role of industry in ensuring safe and efficient use of pesticides: In *Seminar on Safe Handling and Efficient Use of Pesticides.* Kualar Lumpur: Malaysian Agricultural Chemicals Association, 1989.

81. Pesticides Trust. *The FAO Code: Missing Ingredients.* London: Pesticides Trust, 1989.

82. Hurst, P., Dudley, N. and Hay, A. *Pesticides handbook.* Pluto Press, 1991.

83. Watterson A. *Pesticide User's Health and Safety Handbook: An International Guide.* Aldershot: Gower Technical Press, 1989.

84. Mott, L. and Broad, M. *Pesticides in Food.* San Francisco: Natural Resources Defense Council, 1984.

85. Assembly Office of Research. *The Invisible Diet: Gaps in California's Pesticide – Residue Detection Programme.* Sacramento: Assembly Office of Research, 1988.

86. Turnbull, G. J. (ed.) *Occupational Hazards of Pesticide Use.* London: Taylor and Francis, 1985.

87. Matthews, G. A. *Pesticide Application Methods*. London: Longman, 1979.

88. Apple and Pear Development Council. *Orchard and Storage Treatments Used to Combat Fruit Pests and Diseases*. Tunbridge Wells: APDC, 1987.

89. Dudley, N. *Safety Never Assured: An Inquiry into the Practice and Safety of Aerial Spraying*. Stowmarket: Soil Association, 1985.

90. Agricultural Development and Advisory Service. *Aerial Applications Great Britain 1987*. Pesticide usage survey report 72. Alnwick: MAFF, 1988.

91. Environmental Protection Agency. *Report 540/9-75-025*. Washington DC: EPA, 1975.

92. Rose, C. *Pesticides: The First Incidents Report*. London: Friends of the Earth, 1985.

93. Maddy, K. T. and Thomas, W. J. Safe use of pesticides in California, with particular reference to aerial application. *Proceedings of a Symposium on Operational Safety*. ANRC, Canada, 1976.

94. Civil Aviation Authority. *Safety Data Report*. No *Ad Hoc* Vs 026, CAA 1987.

95. *Pesticides Incidents Investigated in 1987* and *Pesticides Incidents Investigated in 1988*. Bootle: Health and Safety Executive, HM Agricultural Inspectorate, 1987, 1988.

96. Egidius, E. and Moster, B. The effects of Neguvon and Nuvan treatment on crabs, lobster and blue mussel. *Agriculture* 1987; **60**, 165–8.

97. World Health Organisation. *Dichlorvos: Environmental Health Criteria*. Geneva: WHO, 1989.

98. Forestry Commission. *Provisional Code of Practice for the Use of Pesticides in Forestry*. Farnham: Forestry Commission, 1989.

99. Health and Safety Commission, Agriculture Industry Advisory Committee. *Paper AIAC 89/6*. HSC, 1989.

100. British Agrochemicals Association. *BAA Amenity Handbook 1990/91*. Peterborough: BAA, 1990.

101. Union of Construction, Allied Trades and Technicians and Transport and General Workers Union. *Pesticides Report*. UCATT/TGWU, 1987.

102. London Hazards Centre. *Toxic Treatments: Wood Preservative Hazards at Work and in the Home*. London: London Hazards Centre, 1989.

103. Rosanove, R. Dangers of the application of lanolin. *Medical Journal of Australia* 1987; **46**, 232.

104. Copeland, C., *et al.* Pesticide residues in lanolin (letter). *Journal of the American Medical Association* 1989; **261**, 242.

105. Dudley, N. Garden chemicals. *Soil Association Quarterly Review* 1986; March, 8–11.

106. British Agrochemicals Association. *Annual Report and Handbook 1988/89*. Peterborough: BAA, 1989.

107. Goulding, R. Poisoning the farm. *Journal of the Society of Occupational Medicine* 1983; **33**, 60–5.

108. Brown, V. K. *Acute Toxicity in Theory and Practice*. Chichester: Wiley, 1980.

109. Proudfoot, A. T. Poisoning treatment centre admissions following acute incidents involving pesticides. *Human Toxicology* 1988; **7**, 255–8.

110. Vale, J. A. *et al*. Acute pesticide poisoning in England and Wales. *Health Trends*. 1987; **19**, 7–5.

111. Department of Health and Social Security. *Pesticide Poisoning: Notes for the Guidance of Medical Practitioners.*.London: HMSO, 1983.

112. Sharp, D. S., *et al*. Delayed health hazards of pesticide exposure. *Annual Review of Public Health* 1986; **7**, 441–71.

113. Cook, R. R., *et al*. Mortality experience of employees exposed to 2,3,7,8-tetrachlorodibenzo-p-dioxin(TCCD). *Journal of Occupational Medicine* 1980; **22**, 530–2.

114. Zack, J. A., and Suskind, R. R. The mortality experience of workers exposed to tetrachlorobenzodioxin in a trichlorophenol processing plant. *Journal of Occupational Medicine* 1980; **22**, 11–14.

115. Ott, M. G., *et al*. A mortality analysis of employees engaged in the manufacture of 2,4,5-trichlorophenoxyacetic acid. *Journal of Occupational Medicine* 1980; **22**, 47–50.

116. Coggon D., *et al*. Mortality of workers exposed to 2 methyl-4-chlorophenoxyacetic acid. *Scandinavian Journal of Work, Environment and Health* 1986; **12**, 448–54.

117. Lynge, E. A follow up study of cancer incidence among workers in the manufacture of phenoxy herbicides in Denmark. *British Journal of Cancer* 1985; **52**, 259–70.

118. Wang, J-D., *et al*. Occupational risk and the development of premalignant skin lesions among paraquat manufacturers. *British Journal of Industrial Medicine* 1987; **44**, 196–200.

119. TGWU, GMB and NUPE. *Pesticides: The Hidden Peril. A Joint TU Report on Pesticide Usage*. London: TGWU/GMB/NUPE, 1986.

120. Health and Safety Executive. *Agricultural Blackspot*. London: HMSO, 1986.

121. Cancer risk of pesticides in agricultural workers: AMA Council on Scientific Affairs Report. *Journal of the American Medical Association* 1988; **260**, 959–66.

122. Saftlas, A. F. Cancer and other causes of death among Wisconsin farmers. *American Journal of Industrial Medicine* 1987; **11**, 119–29.

123. Dubrow, R., *et al*. Farming and malignant lymphoma in Hancock County, Ohio. *British Journal of Industrial Medicine* 1988; **45**, 25–8.

124. Cuzick, J. and de Stavola, B. Multiple Myeloma – a case study. *British Journal of Cancer* 1988; **57**, 516–20.

125. Delzell, E., *et al*. Mortality among white and non white farmers in North Carolina 1976–78. *American Journal of Epidemiology* 1985; **121**, 391–402.

126. Wiklund, K., *et al*. Testicular cancer among agricultural workers and licensed pesticide applicators in Sweden. *Scandinavian Journal of Work Environment and Health* 1986; **12**, 630–31.

127. Blair A. and Thomas, T. L. Leukemia among Nebraska farmers: A death certificate study. *American Journal of Epidemiology* 1979; **110**, 264–73.

128. Burmeister L. F., *et al*. Selected cancer mortality and farm practices in Iowa. *American Journal of Epidemiology* 1983; **118**, 72–7.

129. Burmeister, L. F., *et al*. Leukemia and farm practices in Iowa. *American Journal of Epidemiolology* 1982; **115**, 720–8.
130. Milham, S. Leukemia and multiple myeloma in farmers. *American Journal of Epidemiology* 1971; **94**, 307–10.
131. Priester, W. A. and Mason, T. J. Human cancer mortality in relation to poultry population by county. *Journal of the National Cancer Institute* 1974; **53**, 45–9.
132. Agu, V. U., *et al*. Geographical patterns of multiple myeloma. *Journal of the National Cancer Institute* 1980; **65**, 735–8.
133. Burmeister, L. F. Cancer mortality in Iowa farmers, 1971-8. *Journal of the National Cancer Institute* 1981; **66**, 461–4.
134. Balarajan, R. and Acheson, E. D. Soft tissue sarcomas in agriculture and forestry workers. *Journal of Epidemiology and Community Health* 1984; **38**, 113–6.
135. Buesching, D. and Wollstadt, L. Cancer mortality among farmers. *Journal of the National Cancer Institute* 1984; **72**, 503.
136. Pearce, N. E., *et al*. Malignant lymphoma and multiple myeloma linked with agricultural occupations in a New Zealand cancer registry based study. *American Journal of Epidemiology* 1985; **121**, 225–37.
137. Pearce, N. E., *et al*. Case control study of multiple myeloma and farming. *British Journal of Cancer* 1986; **54**, 493–500.
138. Pearce, N. E., *et al*. Non-Hodgkin's lymphoma and exposure to phenoxy herbicides, chlorophenols, sensing work and meat work employment. *British Journal of Industrial Medicine* 1986; **44**, 75–83.
139. Pearce, N. E., *et al*. Non-Hodgkin's lymphoma and farming: an expanded case control study. *International Journal of Cancer* 1987; **39**, 155–61.
140. Barthel, E. Increased risk of lung cancer in pesticide exposed male agricultural workers. *Journal of Toxicology and Environmental Health* 1981; **8**, 1027–40.
141. Hardell, L. Malignant mesenchymal tumours and exposure to phenoxy acids: a clinical observation. *Lakartidningen* 1977; **74**, 2553–4.
142. Olsson, H. and Brandt, L. Non-Hodgkins lymphoma of the skin and occupational exposure to herbicides. *Lancet* 1981; **ii**, 579.
143. Axelson, O., and Sundell, L. Herbicide exposure, mortality and tumour incidence: an epidemiological investigation on Swedish railroad workers. *Work Environment and Health* 1974; **11**, 21–8.
144. Axelson, O., *et al*. Herbicide exposure and tumour mortality an updated epidemiologic investigation on Swedish railroad workers. *Scandinavian Journal of Work, Environment and Health* 1980; **6**, 73–9.
145. Hardell, L. and Sandstrom, A. Case control study: soft tissue sarcomas and exposure to phenoxyacetic acids or chlorophenols. *British Journal of Cancer* 1979; **39**, 711–17.
146. Hay, A. Phenoxy herbicides, trichlorophenols and soft tissue sarcomas. *Lancet* 1982; **i**, 1240.
147. Hardell, L., *et al*. Malignant lymphoma and exposure to chemicals especially organic solvents, chlorophenols, and phenoxy acids. *British Journal of Cancer* 1981; **43**, 169–76.

148. Hoar, S., *et al.* Agricultural herbicide use and risk of lymphoma and soft-tissue sarcoma. *Journal of the American Medical Association* 1986; **256**, 1141–7.

149. Editorial. Herbicide exposure and cancer. *Journal of the American Medical Association* 1986; **256**, 1176–8.

150. Blair, A., *et al.* Lung cancer and other causes of death among licensed pesticide applicators. *Journal of the National Cancer Institute* 1983; **71**, 31–7.

151. Ott, M. G., *et al.* Respiratory cancer and occupational exposure to arsenicals. *Archives of Environmental Health* 1974; **29**, 250–5.

152. Hardell, L., *et al.* Relation of soft tissue sarcoma, malignant lymphoma, and colon cancer to phenoxy acids, chlorophenols and other agents. *Scandinavian Journal of Work, Environment and Health* 1981; **7**, 119–30.

153. Thiess, A. M., *et al.* Mortality study of persons exposed to dioxin in a trichlorophenol process accident that occurred in the BASF AG on November 17, 1953. *American Journal of Industrial Medicine* 1982; **3**, 179–89.

154. Agent Orange Program. *Mortality Among Vietnam Veterans in Massachusetts, 1972–83.* Boston: Commonwealth of Massachusetts, 1985.

155. Bond, G. C., *et al.* Phenoxy herbicides and cancer: insufficient epidemiological evidence for a causal relationship. *Fundamental and Applied Toxicology* 1989; **12**, 172–88.

156. Carter, R. L. Carcinogenicity of chemicals: the weight of evidence. *Human Toxicology* 1988; **7**, 411–8.

157. Sax, N. I. *Dangerous Properties of Industrial Materials.* New York: Van Nostrand, 1984.

158. Fletcher, A. C. *Reproductive hazards at work.* Manchester: Equal Opportunities Commission, 1985.

159. Hay, A. Defoliants in Vietnam: the long-term effects. *Nature (Lond.)* 1983; **302**, 208-9.

160. Lathrop, G., *et al. An Epidemiological Investigation of Health Effects in Air Force Personnel Following Exposure to Herbicides.* Washington, DC: Surgeon General, 1984.

161. Hatch, M. C. Reproductive effects of the dioxins. In *Public Health Risks of the Dioxins*, William Lowrance (ed.) p. 255–274. Los Altos: Kaufmann, 1984.

162. The Centres for Disease Control Vietnam Experience Study. Health status of Vietnam veterans: reproductive outcomes and child health. *Journal of the American Medical Association* 1988; **259**, 2715–9.

163. Aschengrau, A. and Monson, R. R. Paternal military service in Vietnam and risk of spontaneous abortion. *Journal of Occupational Medicine* 1989; **31**, 618–23.

164. Meselson, M. S., *et al.* Background material to presentation at 1970 American Association for the Advancement of Science Herbicide Assessment Committee. *US Congress Records. 92nd Congress, 2nd Session*, p. 118, 1972.

165. Kunstadter, P. *A Study of Herbicides and Birth Defects in the Republic of Vietnam.* Washington, DC: National Academy of Science, 1982.

166. Procianoy, R. S. Blood pesticide concentrations in mothers and their new born infants. *Acta Paediatrica Scandinavica* 1981; **70**, 925–8.

167. Saxena, M. C., *et al.* Organochlorine pesticides in specimens from women undergoing spontaneous abortion, premature or full term delivery. *Journal of Analytical Toxicology* 1981; **5**, 6–9.

168. Tabershaw, I. R. and Cooper, W. C. Sequelae of acute organophosphate poisoning. *Journal of Occupational Medicine* 1966; **8**, 5–20.

169. Savage, E. P., *et al.* Chronic neurological sequelae of acute organophosphate pesticide poisoning. *Archives of Environmental Health* 1988; **43**, 39–45.

170. Lowengart, R. A., *et al.* Childhood leukaemia and parents' occupational and home exposures. *Journal of the National Cancer Institute* 1987; **79**, 39–46.

171. Weinstein, S. *Fruits of Your Labor: A Guide to Pesticide Hazards for California Field Workers.* Berkeley: University of California, 1984.

172. Abrams, H. K. Case studies in occupational health programs: US–Mexico border industrialisation program. In *Occupational Health and Safety Symposia 1978.* Washington, DC: NIOSH, 1979.

173. World Health Organisation Regional Office for Europe. *Effects of Occupational Factors on Reproduction.* Copenhagen: WHO, 1987.

174. Schwartz, D. A. and Logerfo, J. P. Congenital limb reduction defects in the agricultural setting. *American Journal of Public Health* 1988; **78**, 654–8.

175. MacDonald, A. D., *et al.* Congenital defects and work in pregnancy. *British Journal of Industrial Medicine* 1988; **45**, 581–8.

176. Gordon, J. E. and Shy, C. M. Agricultural chemical use and congenital cleft lip and/or palate. *Archives of Environmental Health* 1981; **36**, 213–21.

177. Kricker, A., *et al.* Women and the environment: a study of congenital limb anomalies. *Community Health Studies* 1986; **10**, 1–11.

178. Balarajan, R and McDowall, M. Congenital malformations and agricultural workers. *Lancet* 1983; **i**, 1112–3.

179. Golding, J. and Sladden, T. Congenital malformations and agricultural workers. *Lancet* 1983; **i**, 1393.

180. Smith, A. H., *et al.* Congenital defects and miscarriages among New Zealand 2,4,5-T sprayers. *Archives of Environmental Health* 1982; **37**, 197–200.

181. Townsend, J. C., *et al.* Survey of reproductive events of wives of employees exposed to chlorinated dioxins. *American Journal of Epidemiology* 1982; **115**, 695–713.

182. Suskind, R. R. and Hertzberg, V. S. Human health effects of 2,4,5-T and its toxic contaminants. *Journal of the American Medical Association* 1984; **251**, 2372–80.

183. Hatch M. C. and Stein, Z. A. Agent Orange and risks to reproduction: the limits of epidemiology. *Teratogenesis, Carcinogenesis and Mutagenesis.* 1986; **6**, 185–202.

184. Luchtrath H. The consequences of chronic arsenic poisoning among Moselle wine growers. *Journal of Cancer Research and Clinical Oncology* 1983; **105**, 173–182.

185. Bartel, E. Increased risk of lung cancer in pesticide exposed male agricultural workers. *Journal of Toxicology and Environmental Health* 1981; **8**, 1027–40.

186. Wiklund K. G., *et al.* Respiratory cancer among orchardists in Washington State 1968-1980. *Journal of Occupational Medicine* 1988; **30**, 561–64.

187. Nelson W. C., *et al.* Mortality among orchard workers exposed to lead arsenate spray: a cohort study. *Journal of Chronic Disease*, 1973; **26**, 105–118.

188. Markovitz, A. and Crosby, W. H. Chemical carcinogenesis: a soil fumigant, 1,3-dichloropropene, as possible cause of hematologic malignancies. *Archives of Internal Medicine* 1984; **144**, 1409–11.

189. Donna A., *et al.* Triazine herbicides and ovarian epithelial neoplasm. *Scandinavian Journal of Work, Environment and Health* 1989; **15**, 47–53.

190. Wang, H. H. and MacMohn, B. Mortality of pesticide applicators. *Journal of Occupational Medicine* 1979; **21**, 741–4.

191. MacMahon, B., *et al.* A second follow-up of mortality in a cohort of pesticide applicators. *Journal of Occupational Medicine* 1988; **30**, 429–32.

192. Morgan E. P., *et al.* Morbidity and mortality in workers occupationally exposed to pesticides. *Archives of Environmental Contamination and Toxicology* 1980; **9**, 349–82.

193. Riihimaki V., *et al.* Mortality of 2,4 dichlorophenoxyacetic acid and 2,4,5 trichlorophenoxyacetic acid herbicide applicators in Finland. *Scandinavian Journal of Work, Environment and Health* 1982; **8**, 37–42.

194. Riihimaki V, *et al.* Mortality and cancer morbidity among chlorinated phenoxy-acid applicators in Finland. *Chemosphere* 1983; **12**, 779–84.

195. Galligher, R. P. and Threlfall, W. J. Cancer and occupational exposure to chlorophenols. *Lancet* 1984; **ii**, 48.

196. Hoar, S. K., *et al.* Agricultural herbicide use and risk of lymphoma and soft tissue sarcoma. *Journal of the American Medical Association* 1986; **256**, 1141–7.

197. Hoar-Zahm, S. K., *et al.* A case referent study of soft tissue sarcoma and Hodgkin's disease. *Scandinavian Journal of Work, Environment and Health* 1988; **14**, 224–30.

198. Wiklund, K., *et al.* Risk of malignant lymphoma in Swedish pesticide appliers. *British Journal of Cancer* 1987; **56**, 505–8.

199. Wiklund, K., *et al.* Risk of malignant lymphoma in Swedish agricultural and forestry workers. *British Journal of Industrial Medicine* 1988; **45**, 19–24.

200. Woods, J. S., *et al.* Soft tissue sarcoma and non-Hodgkin's lymphoma in relation to phenoxyherbicide and chlorinated phenol exposure in Western Washington. *Journal of the National Cancer Institute* 1987; **78**, 899–910.

201. Smith, A. H., *et al.* Soft tissue sarcoma and exposure to phenoxyherbicides and chlorophenols in New Zealand. *Journal of the National Cancer Institute* 1984; **73**, 1111–17.

202. Vineis P, *et al.* Phenoxy herbicides and soft tissue sarcomas in female rice weeders. *Scandinavian Journal of Work, Environment and Health* 1986; **13**, 9–17.

203. Hoar, S. K., *et al.* Herbicides and colon cancer. *Lancet* 1985; **i**, 1277–8.

204. Barthel, E. Retrospective cohort study on cancer frequency in pesticide exposed male pest-control workers. *Zeitschrift fur Erkrangkunfen der Atmung Sorgane* 1986; **166**, 62–8.

205. Cantor, K. P. Farming and mortality from non-Hodgkin's lymphoma: A case control study. *International Journal of Cancer* 1982; **19**, 239–47.

206. Cantor, K. P. and Blair, A. Farming and mortality from multiple meyloma: a case control study with the use of death certificates. *Journal of National Cancer Institute* 1984; **72**, 251–5.

207. Corrao, G., *et al*. Cancer risk in a cohort of licensed pesticide users. *Scandinavian Journal of Work, Environment and Health* 1989; **15**, 203–9.

208. Gallagher, R. P., *et al*. Cancer and plastic anaemia in British Columbia farmers. *Journal of National Cancer Institute* 1984; **72**, 1311–15.

209. Gallagher, R. P., *et al*. Occupational mortality patterns among British Columbia farm workers. *Journal of Occupational Medicine* 1984; **26**, 906–8.

210. Musicco, M., *et al*. Gliomas and occupational exposure to carcinogens: a case control study. *American Journal of Epidemiology* 1982; **116**, 782–90.

211. Musicco, M., *et al*. A case control study of brain gliomas and occupational exposure to chemical carcinogens: the risk to farmers. *American Journal of Epidemiology* 1988; **128**, 778–85.

212. Rafnsson, V. and Gunnarsdottir, H. Mortality among farmers in Iceland. *International Journal of Epidemiology* 1989; **18**, 146–51.

213. Steineck, G. and Wiklund, K. Multiple myelomas in Swedish agricultural workers. *International Journal of Epidemiology* 1986; **15**, 321–5.

214. Wiklund, K., *et al*. Testicular cancer among agricultural workers and licensed pesticide applicators in Sweden. *Scandinavian Journal of Work, Environment and Health* 1986; **12**, 630–1.

215. Wiklund, K., *et al*. Risk of cancer in pesticide applicators in Swedish agriculture. *British Journal of Industrial Medicine* 1989; **46**, 809–14.

216. Atanasov, K., *et al*. Clinical and haematological studies of workers professionally exposed to pesticides. *Folia Medica* 1983; **25**, 35–9.

217. Wang, S., *et al*. Health survey among farmers exposed to deltamethrin in the cotton fields. *Ecotoxicology and Environmental Safety* 1988; **15**, 1–6.

218. Howard, J. K., *et al*. A study of the health of Malaysian plantation workers with particular reference to paraquat spraymen. *British Journal of Industrial Medicine* 1981; **38**, 110–16.

219. Epstein, S. S. and Ozonoff, D. Leukemias and blood dyscrasias following exposure to chlordane and heptachlor. *Teratogenisis, Carcinogenesis and Mutagenesis* 1987; **7**, 527–40.

220. Flodin, U., *et al*. Chronic lymphatic leukaemia and engine exhausts, fresh wood and DDT: a case referent study. *British Journal of Industrial Medicine* 1988; **45**, 33–8.

221. Baker, E. L., *et al.* Epidemic malathion poisoning in Pakistan malaria workers. *Lancet* 1978; **i**, 31–3.

222. Bhy, N., *et al.* Chronic organophosphorus poisoning in pesticide workers. *Indian Journal of Public Health* 1976; **20**, 62–7.

223. Ames, R. G., *et al.* Cholinesterase activity depression among California agricultural pesticide applicators. *American Journal of Industrial Medicine* 1989; **15**, 143–50.

224. Misra, U. K., *et al.* A study of nerve conduction velocity, late responses and neuromuscular synapse function in organophosphate workers in India. *Archives of Toxicology* 1988; **61**, 496–500.

225. Steenland, K., *et al.* Cytogenetic studies in humans after short-term exposure to ethylene dibromide. *Journal of Occupational Medicine* 1985; **27**, 729–32.

226. Rita, P., *et al.* Monitoring of workers occupationally exposed to pesticides in grape gardens in Andhra Pradesh. *Environmental Research* 1987; **44**, 1–5.

227. Maddy, K. T., *et al.* Monitoring the urine of pesticide applicators in California for residues of chlordimeform and its metabolites 1982-1985. *Toxicology Letters (Amsterdam)* 1986; **33**, 37–44.

228. Mathias, C. G. T. and Morrison, J. H. Occupational skin diseases, United States. *Archives of Dermatology (Chicago)* 1988; **124**, 1519–24.

229. Schuman, S. H. and Dodson, R. L. An outbreak of contact dermatitis in farm workers. *Journal of American Academy of Dermatology* 1985; **13**, 220–3.

230. Tucker, S. B. and Flannigan, S. A. Cutaneous effects from occupational exposure to fenvalerate. *Archives of Toxicology* 1983; **54**, 195–202.

231. Seaton, A. The breathless farm worker. *British Medical Journal* 1984; **288**, 1940–1.

232. O'Connell, E. J., *et al.* Childhood hypersensitivity pneumonitis (farmer's lung): four cases in siblings with long term follow-up. *Journal of Pediatrics* 1989; **144**, 995–7.

233. Lings, S. Pesticide lung: a pilot investigation of fruit growers and farmers during the spraying season. *British Journal of Industrial Medicine* 1982; **39**, 370–6.

234. Gerber, W. L., *et al.* Infertility, chemical exposure, and farming in Iowa: absence of an association. *Urology* 1988; **31**, 46–50.

235. Smith, A. H., *et al.* Preliminary report of reproductive outcomes among pesticide applicators using 2,4,5 T. *New Zealand Medical Journal* 1981; **93**, 177–9.

236. Smith, A. H., *et al.* Congenital defects and miscarriages among New Zealand 2,4,5-T sprayers. *Archives of Environmental Health* 1982; **37**, 197–200.

237. Pearn, J. H. Teratogens and the male: an analysis with special reference to herbicide exposure. *Medical Journal of Australia*, 1983; **ii**, 16–20.

238. McDonald, A. D., *et al.* Congenital defects and work in pregnancy. *British Journal of Industrial Medicine* 1988; **45**, 581–8.

239. British Medical Association. *Living With Risk: The BMA Guide.* Chichester: John Wiley 1987. Harmondsworth: Penguin, 1990.

240. Nriagu, J. *Lead and Lead Poisoning*. New York: Wiley Interscience, 1983.

241. Covello, V. T. and Mumpower, J. Risk analysis and risk management: a historical perspective. *Risk Analysis* 1985; **5**, 103.

242. Royal Society Study Group. *Risk Assessment*. London: Royal Society, 1983.

243. Groupement International des Associations Nationales de Fabricants de Produits Agrochimiques. *Carcinogenic Risk Assessment of Pesticides*. Technical monograph, No. 12. Brussels: GIFAP, 1987.

244. Brown, L. P. and Paddle, G. M. Risk assessment: animal or human model? *Pharmaceutical Medicine* 1988; **3**, 361–74.

245. Graham, G. *In Search of Safety: Chemicals and Cancer Risk*. Harvard University Press, 1988.

246. Gilbert, G. N., *et al. Opening Pandora's Box: A Sociological Analysis of Scientists' Discourse*. Cambridge: Cambridge University Press, 1984.

247. Slovic, P., *et al.* Facts and fears: understanding perceived risk. In Schwing, R. C. and Albers, W. A. (eds) *Societal Risk Assessment: How Safe is Safe Enough?* New York: Plenum, 1980.

248. Royal Commission on Environmental Pollution. *Tackling Pollution – Experiences and Prospects* (Cmnd 9149). Tenth Report. London: HMSO, 1984.

249. Johnson, F. R. Economic costs of misinforming about risk: the EDB scare and the media. *Risk Analysis* 1988; **8**, 261–9.

250. Pascoe, D. *Toxicology*. London: Edward Arnold, 1983.

251. Utidjian, H. M. D. The interaction between epidemiology and animal studies in industrial toxicology. In Ballantyne, B. (ed.) *Perspectives in Basic and Applied Toxicology*. London: Wright, 1987.

252. Matsumura, F. *Toxicology of Pesticides*. New York: Plenum, 1975.

253. Bartsch, H. and Malaveille, C. Prevalence of genotoxic chemicals among animal and human carcinogens evaluated in the IARC Monograph series. *Cell Biology and Toxicology* 1989; **5**, 115–27.

254. Chemical Carcinogens: a review of the science and its associated principles by the US Interagency Staff Group on Carcinogens. *Environmental Health Perspectives* 1986; **67**, 201–82.

255. Purchase, I. F. Procedures for screening chemicals for carcinogenicity. *British Journal of Industrial Medicine* 1980; **37**, 1–10.

256. Hay, A. How to identify a carcinogen. *Nature (Lond.)* 1988; **332**, 782–3.

257. Ames, B., *et al.* Ranking possible carcinogenic hazards. *Science* 1987; **236**, 271–80.

258. Epstein, S. S. and Schwartz, J. B. Carcinogenic risk estimation. *Science* 1988; **240**, 1043–7.

259. BMA and Faculty of Community Medicine. *The State of Community Medicine*. London: BMA, 1979.

260. Hawkins, L. *Planning for Health: The Information Needs of Community Medicine*. Southampton: Health Compass, 1986.

261. Tomenson, J. A. and Brown, L. P. Epidemiology in relation to toxicology. In Marrs, T., Turner, P. and Balantyne, B. (eds) *A Textbook of Basic and Applied Toxicology*. Macmillan, London, 1991.

262. Health Services Information Steering Group. *Converting Data into Information*. London: Kings Fund, 1982.

263. Vale, J. A., *et al*. Acute pesticide poisoning in England and Wales. *Health Trends* 1987; **19**, 5–7.

264. Ministry of Agriculture, Fisheries and Food. Agricultural Science (1985–86). MAFF, 1987.

265. Ministry of Agriculture Fisheries and Food. *Report of the Working Party on Pesticide Residues 1985–88*. Surveillance Paper No.25. London: HMSO, 1989.

266. Home Grown Cereals Authority. *The Occurrence and Detection of Pesticide Residues in UK Grain*. London: HGCA, 1989.

267. British Agrochemicals Association. *Pesticide Residues and Water*. Peterborough: BAA, 1988.

268. World Health Organisation. *Drinking Water Quality: Guidelines for Selected Herbicides*. Environmental Health No.27. Geneva: WHO, 1987.

269. Natural Resources Defense Council. *Intolerable Risk: Pesticides in our Children's Food*. Washington, DC: NRDC, 1989.

270. Jensen, A. A. Chemical contaminants in human milk. *Residue Review* 1983; **89**, 1–128.

271. Chemical residues in food. *Lancet* 1989; **i**, 1009–10.

272. Alar withdrawn in US. *Lancet* 1989; **i**, 1463.

273. Wilkinson, C. F. and Ginevan, M. E. *A Critical Review of the Natural Resources Defense Council's Report 'Intolerable Risk: Pesticides in our Children's Food'*. Springfield, USA: Risk Focus, 1989.

274. Ministry of Agriculture, Fisheries and Food. *Investigations of Suspected Poisoning of Animals by Pesticides in Great Britain 1985–7*. Report of the Environmental Panel on the Advisory Committee on Pesticides. London: MAFF, 1989.

275. Sheail, J. *Pesticides and Nature Conservation: The British Experience 1950–75*. Oxford: Clarendon Press, 1985.

276. Institute of Biology. *Britain Since 'Silent Spring': An Update on the Ecological Effects of Agricultural Pesticides in the UK*. London: Institute of Biology, 1988.

277. Institute of Biology. *Ecotoxicology: Proceedings of a Joint Symposium of the Institute of Biology and the British Toxicological Society*. London: Institute of Biology, 1989.

278. British Agrochemical Association. *The Plain Man's Guide to the New Pesticide Regulations*. Peterborough: BAA, 1987.

279. *Pesticides 1988: Pesticides Approved Under the Control of Pesticides Regulations 1986*. MAFF Reference Book 500. London: HMSO, 1988.

280. Wingfield, J. Controls on pesticides and other substances hazardous to health. *Pharmaceutical Journal* **17 Dec**, 784, 1988.

281. Ministry of Agriculture, Fisheries and Food. *Revised Draft Storage Code of Practice*. Alnwick: Pesticides Safety Division, MAFF, 1988.

282. Ministry of Agriculture, Fisheries and Food and the Health and Safety Commission. *Pesticides: Code of Practice for the Safe Use of Pesticides on Farms and Holdings.* London: HMSO, 1990.

283. Jabbari, D. Food contamination from additives and pesticide residues. *Law Society's Gazette* 1988; **34**, 21–5.

284. World Health Organisation Regional Office for Europe. *Health and the Environment.* Copenhagen: WHO, 1986.

285. UNEP/FAO/WHO. *Guidelines for Predicting Dietary Intake of Pesticide Residues.* Geneva: WHO, 1989.

286. Department of the Environment Central Directorate of Environmental Protection. *Report on an Inter-Departmental Working Party on Public Access to Information held by Pollution Control Authorities.* Pollution Paper No. 23. London: HMSO, 1986

287. Rowell, R. *Practical Food Law Manual.* London: Sweet and Maxwell, 1988.

288. Dayan, A. D. Who needs toxicology? *Journal of the Royal Society of Medicine* 1989; **82**, 320–1.

289. Jackson J. R. *Attributes and Teaching Relative to Pesticides in British Medical Schools* (unpublished observations).

290. Jones, J. S. Responses to chemical warfare. *Nature (Lond.)* 1989; **337**, 690.

291. Gunn, D. L. Alternatives to chemical pesticides. In Gunn, D. L. and Stevens, J. G. R. (eds) *Pesticides and Human Welfare.* 241–55 Oxford: Oxford University Press, 1976.

292. Huffaker, C. B. Biological control. In *Proceedings of American Association for the Advancement of Science Symposium, Boston, December 1969.* New York: Plenum, 1971.

293. Price Jones, D. and Solomon, M. E. *Biology in Pest and Disease Control. 13th Symposium of the British Ecological Society, Oxford, 1972.* Oxford: Blackwell, 1974.

294. Van den Bosch, R. *The Pesticide Conspiracy.* Dorchester: Prism, 1980.

295. Alexander, R. and Anderson, P. K. Pesticide use, alternatives and workers' health in Cuba. *International Journal of Health Services* 1984; **14**, 31–41.

296. Swezey, S. L., *et al. Getting off the Pesticides Treadmill in the Developing World: Nicaragua's Revolution in Pesticide Policy.* Leon: University of Nicaragua, 1984.

297. Dover, M. J. *A Better Mousetrap: Improving Pest Management for Agriculture.* Washington, DC: World Resources Institute, 1985.

298. Pesticides Action Network. *Fighting Pests the Natural Way: An Introduction to the Protection of Plants without Synthetic Pesticides.* Brussels: PAN, 1988.

299. American Council on Science and Health. *Pesticides: Helpful or Harmful?* New York: ACSH, 1988.

300. Richards, P. *Indigenous Agricultural Revolution.* London: Hutchinson, 1985.

301. Greig-Smith P. W. The Boxworth Project – Environmental Effects of Cereal Pesticides. *Journal of the Royal Agricultural Society* 1989; **150**, 171–87.

302. *House of Lords Science and Technology Report.* Fifth Report 1984. *Agricultural and Environmental Research.* London: HMSO, 1984.

303. *Government Response to the Fifth Report of the House of Lords Science and Technology Report 1984–5.* London: HMSO, 1985.

304. King, E. G. Potential for biological control of Heliothis species. *Annual Review of Entomology* 1989; **34**, 53–75.

305. Debach, P. and Schlinger, E. J. *Biological Control of Insect Pest and Weeds.* London: Chapman and Hall, 1964.

306. Caltagirone, L. E. and Doutt, R. L. The history of vedalia beetle importation to California and its impact on the development of biological control. *Annual Review of Entomology* 1989; **34**, 1–16.

307. Taylor, T. H. C. Biological control of insect pests. *Annals of Applied Biology* 1955; **42**, 190–6.

308. Hansen, M. *Escape from the Pesticide Treadmill.* Penang: International Organisation of Consumers Unions Pesticide Action Network, 1987.

309. Argov, Y. and Rossler, Y. Introduction of beneficial insects into Israel for the control of insect pests. *Phytoparasitica* 1988; **16**, 303–15.

310. Burges, H. D. and Hussey, N. W. *Microbial Control of Insects and Mites.* London: Academic Press, 1971.

311. Franz, J. M. and Krieg, A. *Biologische Schadlingsbekampfung* 3rd edn. Berlin: Paul Parey, 1982.

312. Campion, D. G. Survey of pheromone uses in pest control. In Hummel, H. E. and Miller, T. A. (eds) *Techniques in Pheromone Research*, p. 405–99. New York: Springer Verlag, 1984.

313. Jones, O. T. Chemical mediation of insect behaviour. In Hutson, D. H. and Roberts, T. R. (eds) *Insecticides.* Chichester: John Wiley, pp.311–73, 1985.

314. Wall, C. Application of sex attractants for monitoring the pea moth, *Cydia nigricana* (F) (*Lepidoptera: Tortricidae*). *Journal of Chemical Ecology* 1988; **14**, 1855–64.

315. Pickett, J. A. The future of semiochemicals in pest control. *Aspects of Applied Biology* 1988; **17**, 397–406.

316. Debach, P. *Biological Control by Natural Enemies.* Cambridge: Cambridge University Press, 1974.

317. Sun, M. Preparing the ground for biotech tests. *Science* 1988; **242**, 503–5.

318. McGaughey, W. H. Insect resistance to the biological insecticide *Bacillus thuringiensis. Science* 1985; **229**, 193–5.

319. Davidson, G. *Genetic Control of Insect Pests.* London: Academic Press, 1974.

320. Royal Commission on Environmental Pollution. Thirteenth Report. *The Release of Genetically Engineered Organisms to the Environment* (Cmnd 720). London: HMSO, 1989.

321. National Academy of Sciences. *Alternative Agriculture.* Washington, DC: NAS 1989.

322. Association of London Chief Environmental Health Officers. *A Report on a London-wide Survey of Drinking Water Quality.* Chelmsford: Berridge Environmental Laboratories, 1990.

323. *This Common Inheritance: Britain's Environmental Strategy.* (Cm 1200). London: HMSO, 1990.

324. Ministry of Agriculture, Fisheries and Food (1990). *Food labelling survey of England and Wales – Report on a survey carried out in April and May 1990.* London: HMSO, 1990.

INDEX

023991